TOXIC Chemical-Free Living

AND RECOVERING FROM ME/CFS

Trixie Whitmore

SALLY MILNER PUBLISHING

First published in 1990 by
Sally Milner Publishing Pty Ltd
17 Wharf Road
Birchgrove NSW 2041 Australia

Reprinted 1990, 1991

©Trixie Whitmore 1990
Production by Sylvana Scannapiego, Island Graphics
Cover design by Elaine Rushbrooke
Photography by Russell Cockayne and John Wilcock
Photographer's model Elizabeth Hamilton
Typeset in 11/13pt Goudy Old Style by
Trade Graphics Pty Ltd, Melbourne
Printed in Australia by
Australian Print Group

National Library of Australia
Cataloguing-in-Publication data:

Whitmore, Trixie.
   Toxic chemical-free living and recovery from ME/CFS

   ISBN 1 86351 000 1.

   1. Myalgic encephalomyelitis. 2. Chronic fatigue syndrome.
   3. Chemicals — Physiological effect. I. Title.

616.74

Distributed in Australia and New Zealand exclusively by
Transworld Publishers

Front cover:
Moonrise Heidelberg 1900
Emmanuel Phillips Fox 1865–1915
oil on canvas, 75.8 x 126.5 cm
Purchased 1948
National Gallery of Victoria

This book is user friendly. It:
is printed on **RE△RIGHT** 100% Re-cycled Paper;
is bound with glue which contains no formaldehyde,
no petrochemicals and no aromatic solvents;
is 100% Australian.

Foreword

Trixie was my first ME/CFS case. She presented as such. When I positioned her for the gentle thrust of the manipulation, instead of the usual 'click' that I expected, she reacted by going into muscle spasm. I massaged her out of that, but was intrigued by the different 'feel' of her muscles. Her proposed medical practitioner, Dr Eric, was well-known to me and highly respected for his expert diagnosis and his open-mindedness. I certainly wished to be kept informed of this unusual case. She had chosen correctly, as Dr Eric had already become very familiar with ME/CFS cases.

Trixie reacts very quickly. When I used baby oil on her it burnt her skin. We quickly realised only pure vegetable oils such as olive oil, apricot oil, grape oil etc. could be used on her skin. I have subsequently found this to be so with all my ME/CFS cases.

I continue to help Trixie within my expertise and find muscle manipulation and acupuncture, together with a diet of non-allergenic foods and homoeopathy, to be responsible for her recovery — not forgetting of course her indomitable courage and sheer strength of will that never let her down when her hostile environment did.

This is her story and I recommend it to those who suffer from this debilitating condition and are looking for practical help.

This book will provide many answers to problems. It is also a warning to the people of the world that our environment has now turned hostile owing to man's greed, the irresponsibility of many companies and to our apathy.

Leonie McMahon

Dear Reader

At last someone is prepared to look at a possible toxic chemical connection with ME/CFS. Dr Tapen Mukherjee of the Adelaide Institute of Medical and Veterinary Sciences, with the assistance of the South Australian Government, has purchased equipment and set up a research unit to investigate the possible causes of ME/CFS.

Mukherjee is anxious to engage a toxicologist to work along with him, therefore I am hoping that the proceeds from my share (10%) of the book will be sufficient to make a donation towards his research.

If you know anyone interested in donating to this research, monies can be sent to: —

ME SOCIETY OF SOUTH AUSTRALIA
GPO BOX 383
ADELAIDE 5001.

A special trust account has been opened by the ME Society at the Adelaide University for all donations to Dr Mukherjee's research.

I am at present trying to get some corporate sponsorship for this important research. If you have any contacts with companies who might be prepared to assist in any way financially either follow it up yourself or let me know about it.

We must find out the *cause* of our illness! Scientifically!

Trixie Whitmore.

Contents

Acknowledgements

I dedicate this book to my husband, Paul, without whom I could not have persevered through my relapses and long periods of recovery. He has shown the kindness, patience and consideration few men possess. There is no doubt that without family support I would not have made such a succession of recoveries. He has been the breadwinner, the nurse, the cook and cleaner; he has sorted out the children and seen to all their needs. He has dropped everything to take me to Dr Eric or Leonie McMahon when I could barely walk, and though I was and looked a complete wreck of a woman, he has never stopped loving and caring for me. That takes a very special person.

Over the years the children have come to an understanding of my problems; with maturity they, too, have shown love and caring, and I am so very proud of each one of them.

To my only daughter I say a special thank you for her wonderful love and understanding.

Thank you Paul, Elizabeth, David, John, Tony and Greg.

I owe a debt of gratitude to Leonie McMahon, registered chiropractor, osteopath and qualified homoeopath, acupuncturist and ortho-molecular nutritionist. She persuaded me (with some difficulty) to write my story, in the hope that it may in some way alleviate suffering and help restore health to those unfortunate enough to fall victim of

ME/CFS. I was encouraged to do so also by my doctor, Dr Eric MB, BS, FRACGP, homoeopath, acupuncturist, education officer for the Australian Medical Faculty of Homoeopathy. Both of these practitioners have been a source of inspiration, encouragement and practical help during the years I have battled to get back on my feet. I can never thank them enough for their caring and kindness and for their skills — they are practitioners rarely found in these days of regimented medicine, who take a real interest in each and every patient who passes through their doors. They both possess open minds and will look much further than the basic principles of conventional medicine and the narrow paths they were initially taught to follow. They have a range of skills in what is classified as 'alternative medicine' and, combined with their conventional allopathic skills, they are the practitioners of the future. This is borne out by the results they achieve and the satisfaction of their patients.

I will never be able to sufficiently express my gratitude to Leonie or Dr Eric — suffice it to say that I have made two quite wonderful friends.

I would also like to give thanks to my dentist, Dr R. (Ron) Ehrlich, who kindly consulted with Dr Eric as to my sensitivities and has gone to a lot of trouble to use products which do not cause me any harm. He also is a forward thinking, open-minded, highly skilled practitioner, who is constantly improving his range of skills.

I have contacted many manufacturers during the course of my investigations and found them to be more than helpful, to be pretty honest about the pitfalls of some of their products and to be very amenable to the idea of taking a closer look to improve the safety, non-allergenic qualities and disposability of their products. This is very encouraging. In particular, I would like to thank:

Lever and Kitchen (manufacturers of Sunlight and Velvet

soaps and soap powders) for the interest they took on behalf of myself and other sensitive people.

Glenys Lord, Marketing Consultant to Herbonics, Australia, for the help they gave me in the production of my book. I have been using their soap, detergent, shampoo and dishwashing powder for the last year or two and have found them excellent. They have recently added new products to their range.

Dekris Pty Ltd of Caringbah, New South Wales, for donating the 'Cellophane' bags to the ME Society of New South Wales for wrapping.

Alliance Packaging of Revesby, New South Wales for donating the cardboard boxes to the ME Society.

Lynne Field of ACL Films, Victoria. Lynne went to no end of trouble to give me truthful information about the 'Cellophane' food wrapping, and through her contacts I was able to organise wrapping and packaging for the charcoal masks (see page 159). She also kindly sent me a roll of 'Cellophane' film to try out.

3M Australia Pty Ltd for its generous ongoing donation of masks to the ME Society of New South Wales.

The Total Environment Centre and Systems Pest Management, who were caring and helpful.

National Health and Medical Research Council; CSIRO; NSW Division of Occupational Health; Workers' Compensation and Rehabilitation Authority for their assistance and constant supply of information.

Preface

This is my story and, except where otherwise stated, the opinions in this book are my own and have been formed because of my own experience and research.

In 1983 I was struck down with Myalgic Encephalomyelitis (ME) which is also known as Chronic Fatigue Syndrome (CFS). It has been called 'Yuppie Flu'. It is one of the most devastating and frustrating illnesses for it does not fall into a definite 'clinical diagnosis' and no one can really understand its effects unless they have suffered from it themselves.

This book is an account of the treatments I explored, the ones I found to be of great benefit to myself, and my discovery of what had made me sick in the first place. I experienced three very severe relapses which totally incapacitated me for a considerable period of time, and this is the story of what I did to regain my health. It may be of benefit to anyone suffering from this syndrome or to those who know someone who is suffering. I hope it will be of benefit to the medical profession at large as it is a patient's point of view, sometimes very much overlooked.

It is also a warning to everyone that the world we have taken for granted has now turned hostile — you could be the next victim! It's important for us to clean up our own environment and in doing so we will reap the rewards of better health as well as helping to alleviate the pollution of our world.

Read these pages and you will see that there *are* safe alternatives to toxic chemicals which are destroying our world and making us ill. Do your bit for the environment. Show an example. Then make industry and agriculture clean up their act by boycotting toxic products and demanding clean air, clean water and clean food — necessities which are almost lost if we do not act now.

I   *Understanding the illness*

1   ME/CFS: Symptoms, causes, diagnosis and recovery

ME/CFS is the abnormal response of the body to either a virus or some other trigger factor which leaves the person in a constant state of fatigue and malaise. It is known to have occurred after:
- a severe virus or infection
- innoculations
- exposure to certain toxic chemicals (including drugs).

Other people have progessed slowly into the syndrome over a period of years with no apparent trigger factor.

Many people suffer what is called Post Viral Fatigue following glandular fever, hepatitis, influenza, etc. when their body demands much more rest than normal and when they simply do not feel 'well'. If they look after themselves and have plenty of rest, they usually recover after three to six months.

However, it is when the fatigue and feeling of malaise continues, is exacerbated by exercise, and other symptoms develop that a diagnosis of ME/CFS can be suspected.

Symptoms

I have noted on the following pages all the symptoms I experienced with ME/CFS.

As we are all individuals do not be alarmed if your own particular symptoms are not mentioned. I can only identify the ones I have experienced. However, many are common symptoms experienced by most people with ME/CFS. It's important to remember that these may be symptoms with which anyone can identify, as they may also indicate allergies and/or sensitivities which will be discussed later.

General debilitation
- complete and absolute exhaustion
- body feels like lead and is sinking through mattress
- effort to speak let alone move
- cannot get warm
- so ill thought I was dying
- loss of vitality

Circulation
- burning just under skin which feels like burning hot ice, and pins and needles at the same time
- arms and legs burn with cold, and elbows and knees cold to touch
- loss of circulation in feet and hands

Limbs and muscles
- vibrations of parts of or entire body upon movement
- 'motor' running in legs
- trembling muscles
- stabbing pains in various parts of the body, especially arms and legs
- sore feet
- pain in back, shoulders and neck, lower back, hips and ankles
- sprained ribs
- muscles tied up in knots
- cramps
- great soreness of joints (wrist in splint at one stage)

Eyes
- loss of eye function
- sore and bloodshot eyes
- watery eyes when watching TV or reading
- cannot hold up eyelids
- huge black circles around eyes in deathly white face

Ears, nose, throat and chest
- ringing in ears
- very thirsty
- sore throat
- sore nose with pustules and breakdown of mucous membranes
- itching of nose and chin
- catarrh
- earache
- thrush of mouth
- shortness of breath and wheezing
- constriction of throat and chest
- tachycardia (palpitations)

Digestive system
- nausea
- sick feeling in pit of stomach
- indigestion and upset bowel
- thrush of colon
- bloated stomach
- acute pain and cramps in bowel
- diarrhoea and foamy stools
- loss of control of bowel and bladder

Psychological state
- inability to cope with slightest stress
- inability to concentrate
- forgetfulness

- very depressed
- very agitated — nerves seem to be banging against each other, cannot relax
- mood swings

Other

- vertigo (dizziness)
- headaches
- thrush of vagina and breakdown of mucous membranes
- allergies to various foods and chemicals
- swollen glands
- hot and cold sweats and hot flushes
- sleeplessness
- sores on lips and vagina
- bruising at slightest bump
- rashes

Causes of ME/CFS

There are two main schools of thought as to the cause of ME/CFS. Neither has as yet been proven.

First, *a severe virus or infection is suspected of being the cause.* Glandular fever, influenza, hepatitis seem to be the most common ones. This leads in some way to a debilitated immune system and the body never seems to completely recover. Thus one becomes very allergic to various foods and chemicals which cause the body to relapse into a post-viral syndrome of fatigue and malaise. Some of the people Dr Eric and I have questioned seem to have developed the syndrome very gradually, over a period of years, and a particular virus does not seem to have been the trigger. Why do some people recover completely from these viruses and not other people? Also, why is it not one particular virus as is the case with AIDS? That is the puzzle.

Professor John Dwyer and Professor Denis Wakefield have

done an enormous amount of clinical research into ME/CFS at Sydney's Prince of Wales and Prince Henry Hospitals. They have treated people with gamma-globulin serum and transfer factor to try to boost the immune system. This has resulted in an improvement in some patients, but has had no beneficial effects on others. They have researched viruses and the immune system and their research has benefited enormously from their own findings as to how the immune system works (Professor Wakefield's report to the ME Society, January 1989). It is thanks to the tremendous efforts of the ME Society that this research was even begun, as only a few years ago the ME Society was just a small bunch of sick people trying to get someone to listen to them. Now they have achieved some government assistance, but need lots more as many more people are stricken with the illness.

Second, there is another school of thought being investigated by other doctors, *that reactions to, and/or overload of toxic chemicals are the cause rather than the effect of ME/CFS.* This theory is built on the premise that many drugs and toxic chemicals are known to deplete or damage the immune system, thus rendering it unable to fight and recover from a severe virus, or even a mild virus or infection. It may be that a combination of some or all of the following, causes an overload situation, or permanent damage to the immune system:

- antibiotics, antibacterial and other drugs
- steroids (eg cortisone)
- the contraceptive pill
- innoculations and vaccinations (by altering the T-cell balance)
- transfusion reaction
- toxic chemicals, particularly pesticides and herbicides and volatile aromatic and chlorinated solvents
- viruses and infections.

I must say that I subscribe to this theory of a

debilitated immune system because of toxic chemicals in the environment. It seems logical when an investigation is made of the toxic effects of many products freely available on the market today and it would make sense for toxicologists to be working along with the professors doing all this wonderful work. The symptoms of pesticide poisoning are synonymous with the symptoms of ME/CFS.

Why do some people get ME/CFS and others don't? Why do some people get cancer, asthma, Parkinson's disease, Alzheimer's disease? These are also known or suspected to be caused by toxic chemicals. For example, cigarette smoke can cause cancer because of the toxic chemicals contained in the smoke. Obviously we are all being affected by the toxicity in our environment but it is manifesting itself in different people in different ways. It would be interesting to investigate the DNA of all ME/CFS sufferers to see if there is a common link making them more susceptible genetically to this breakdown. (This has proven to be the case in some rheumatoid arthritis sufferers who share a common DNA factor.) Conversely, it may be that the levels of one or more toxic chemicals in ME/CFS sufferers are the culprit. Also, what effect would a 'cocktail' of toxic chemicals have on the metabolism? Chemicals can react with each other. Was enough care taken in this regard before certain drugs and chemicals were released onto the market?

Another interesting discovery regarding ME/CFS was by Dr Tapen M. Mukherjee (MBBS, MD, FRCPA, Head of Electron Microscopy and Clinical Senior Lecturer in Pathology at the Institute of Medical and Veterinary Science at Adelaide University). When investigating the blood of ME/CFS patients in relapse he found that the red blood cells became deformed, changed shape, and consequently did not flow through the small capillaries easily. Deformities of red blood cells were also observed by Professor John A. Sirs of the Department of Physiology and Biophysics at St Mary's Hospital Medical School, University of London, during and after cardiac bypass surgery. He passed these observations on to Dr Mukherjee who commented, in a personal communication to me,

> It was interesting to note how the ME/CFS blood showed transient deformation of red blood cells as was also observed by Professor Sirs in cases of cardiac bypass surgery patients. While discussing the relationship between the two completely unrelated situations the question of the anaesthetics applied during the surgical procedures came into consideration and seemed likely to be the source of such deformations of the red blood cells. Anaesthetics are known to be toxic to certain persons and that raises the question — could they be responsible for the red blood cell deformations observed in a variety of conditions?

Dr Mackarness in his book *Chemical Victims* says that the anaesthetics and the fumes from the heart/lung machine contributed to a colleague's illness which occurred in the operating theatre (dizziness, headache and flu-like symptoms). Could there be some significance in these similarities? After all, anaesthethics are toxic chemicals!

It is also interesting to note that many sufferers are thin people. Could it be that thin people do not have enough fatty tissue to store these toxic chemicals?

One GP I met at a seminar commented to me that most of his ME/CFS patients were 'A' type personalities, i.e. they had led vital and challenging lives, were high achievers and were not the types of people to suddenly be classified as neurotic. Dr Eric verifies this.

Another interesting phenomenon I have noticed is the fact that during the latter months of pregnancy ME/CFS sufferers seem to look and feel much better. It is a theory of mine that toxic chemicals may have either destroyed or affected the production of certain bacteria, enzymes or hormones in our bodies, thus upsetting the delicate balance of nature.

Is it possible that these essential enzymes or hormones are produced by a growing foetus and circulated in the blood of the mother, improving her condition?

Dr Eric and I undertook some basic research to see if ME/CFS patients had reactions similar to mine when exposed to chemicals. While it was not a properly conducted scientific experiment, the results supported many of the conclusions I have made. The questionnaire we sent out and the results are in Further Information (page 201).

Diagnosis and recovery

The effect of any disease will vary with individuals because each of us has a different DNA (except in the case of identical twins). Therefore with our differing metabolisms we must expect each person to have individual reactions to almost everything. No two people who get stomach cancer, for example, have exactly the same symptoms, nor does the disease follow exactly the same pattern. Asthma would be another example. Much depends on the mental and physical make-up of each person as to how that illness will affect them. That is one of the weaknesses of modern medicine. Illnesses are usually categorised, presumed to follow a set pattern, and treated accordingly, with minimal consideration of the individual concerned.

ME/CFS is a good example of this. It has taken years for anyone even to recognise that it exists as it does not respond to a standard blood test. I have a close friend who at the age of eighteen was rushed to hospital with suspected heart trouble when she experienced palpitations (tachycardia) and pain rushing up to her neck and down her left arm. She had been feeling very tired at the time. She was discharged from hospital as nothing abnormal could be found. She progressed into a state of malaise and depression and looked like death. She lost weight and could barely walk without her heart palpitating. She had huge black circles under her eyes, her neck glands were swollen, her face was as white as a sheet and on referral to one specialist after another (where she would break down and cry because she was getting nowhere) was constantly told she was neurotic and needed Valium. Thank goodness her family had faith in the fact that she had previously been a very independent and happy young woman and they refused to believe she could change so dramatically overnight. This was many years ago when ME/CFS was virtually undiagnosed. Anyone can understand the effect all this had on her mentality. She became frightened, the palpitations turned to panic attacks and she ended up with agoraphobia. This is not unusual in ME/CFS cases as is now evident. Many more sick people have no doubt been treated in this way, all because their symptoms do not fit a 'clinical pattern'. In the end she consulted a chiropractor who thought she had been affected by a virus, prescribed lots of vitamin C and did her more good than anyone else. He certainly did not tell her she was neurotic.

The most important factor in coping with any illness, and particularly ME/CFS, is to find a practitioner who is understanding and who has an open mind, because the malady does not seem to respond well to conventional medicine. The other most important factor is to remember that one cannot just bundle up an illness and drop it in the doctor's lap for him or her to solve. Each and everyone of us must take responsibility for our illnesses and do as much as we can in all the hours of convalescing to find out what will help us personally, to avoid that which does not, and to adopt the most positive attitude towards healing.

Recovery rates from ME/CFS seem to conform to three patterns:

1 Some patients recover completely after about six to twelve months, or longer.
2 Some patients follow a pattern of recovery and relapse.

(I know of cases where people have recovered completely within twelve months and years later suffered a severe and continuing relapse.)
3 Other cases become chronic and may be partially or completely invalided.

I commented to Dr Eric last year that it seemed to me that the patient contributed about 65 per cent towards their cure and the doctor 35 per cent. He corrected me and said 'Rather, Trixie, 90 per cent patient, 10 per cent doctor'. He is a realist and unlike most doctors talks to me as though I am an intelligent person. He listens to me, discusses and explains everything to me, has an open mind, encourages me to try new and different approaches and believes that the patient cannot be chopped up into little pieces, but must be treated as a whole person, with the spirit, the mind and the body all at peace within that person — how logical this seems.

2   A brief history of illness: my story

I will sketch briefly the circumstances of my illness in the hope that some, or all of it, might be helpful to ME/CFS sufferers and as an example to anyone not familiar with ME/CFS who might be interested in learning more about it.

Prior to June 1983 I had, for some twelve months or more, been suffering from muscle tiredness, shortness of breath, dry and sore nose and throat, bleeding nose, catarrh and sinus/rhinitis. Some of these symptoms worsened when I mowed the lawn with our 2 stroke mower. A series of routine allergy tests at Royal North Shore Hospital showed virtually nothing. The shortness of breath persisted, I began to wheeze and had to give up playing squash. I also noticed that certain smells, particularly petrol fumes and cigarette smoke, were annoying me although I paid little attention at the time.

I was under a good deal of stress at home. I had remarried in 1981 and the last and youngest of our combined tribe of five had decided to move in with the rest of our mob; so I acquired a strong-willed, fifteen year-old lad and there began a battle of wills between us. Anyone who has reared teenage boys can understand the difficulties. However, I am happy to say that he and I are now the greatest of friends. Nevertheless, I make mention of this to illustrate that I was not living in what could be described as 'a peaceful environment' — hardly, with five children between the ages of twenty-three and fifteen and a reasonably new husband!

Over the years I had been exposed unwittingly to many toxic chemicals. I had used creosote stains, Estapol, paints, glues, polishes, wood stains and solvents, as we had built a house in 1968 (which was treated for white ants with dieldrin) and had done a great deal of the work ourselves, expecially the painting and staining. The house had polished floors which required the application of mineral turpentine (turps) and wax to keep them in good order. I used napthalene liberally in the cupboards and on the rugs and floors, as we had a cat which seemed to encourage periodic outbreaks of fleas. About this time I was persuaded to use Baygon (I have always been very wary of poisons) as the fleas were persistent. We also lived alongside a golf course and at times various very strong smells wafted into our home following the treatments of the fairways and greens.

In late June we went for a skiing holiday to Smiggins in the Snowy Mountains of New South Wales. While there I contracted a viral influenza which became known as 'the Philippine Flu'. I was extremely ill for some weeks, had difficulty breathing and was treated by the local doctor with penicillin. This was against my better judgement as I had previously suffered side-effects, including thrush (candida), on the few occasions I had taken antibiotics. At the time I became ill I had sprinkled napthalene extensively over the carpet of the bedroom to counter the fleas. The smell was most unpleasant and worried me, although I had used it for years.

After about five weeks I recovered and with the doctor's permission returned to the ski fields, this time to a private lodge in the Snowy Mountains. We spent a week there, but I was not managing to ski well as my legs seemed unable to control my skis. (My husband says I must mention here that I blamed my boots, my skis, my stocks — everything except my legs — for not being able to ski properly.)

I was also having breathing difficulties whilst in the lodge.

The managers of the lodge applied a carpet deodoriser each week and the smell was really causing me to suffer. The smell was so overpowering I found it difficult to sleep at night, and I would find myself standing at the open window (it was zero degrees outside) taking gasps of icy cold air to relieve my breathlessness. My throat was sore too, although no cold symptoms eventuated.

First ME/CFS Attack

Back home again, after returning everything to order and polishing the floor with mineral turps and wax, I remember standing at the stove cooking dinner, noticing the smell of the turps fumes burning as well. I was overwhelmed with the most dreadful sick feeling and found myself the next day with a relapse of the 'flu'. Although I had no temperature, I experienced the most profound weakness and feeling of incredible illness. I was afraid to sleep as I was constantly suffocating and I had to keep a hotpot of boiling water beside my bed to help my breathing.

The local doctor prescribed more penicillin, and although I was reluctant to take it, he said it was absolutely necessary and I think I felt so ill I would have swallowed anything in the hope of recovery. However, I developed severe thrush and I just seemed to get worse and worse and finally my leg muscles went into spasms. I thought I had polio. At this stage I had been in bed for two months. My weight was 40kg (6 stone 4lbs).

I was then referred to a physician who gave me a complete checkup, including blood tests. He could not find anything physically amiss and said I had had a severe virus which seemed to have affected the nervous system and that I would eventually recover.

I did eventually improve, although I did not recover my previous health. My body felt tied up in knots, my back and chest were so tight and sore, my legs were tired and sore, I was constantly fatigued and could not sleep.

One of my sons decided 'Mum was just not fit' and advised that I start exercising on the exercise bike to rebuild my muscles. This was disastrous. After five minutes my legs completely collapsed and I was helped to bed where I stayed for some days before I could walk again.

In early January 1984 I went to the country to help a friend with a wedding. This proved too much for me and I relapsed. By the end of January I was virtually dragging myself around and the local doctor did not know what was wrong with me. I mentioned this to an old friend of mine who is in her eighties. She recommended that I contact her doctor, who is also a homoeopath, and who had effected some wonderful cures in her family over the years. Unfortunately he was booked up for six months so I was referred to his partner, Dr Eric, who could see me in two weeks' time.

A few days later, whilst making the effort to shop at West Lindfield, I encountered another friend who said she was visiting her chiropractor, Leonie McMahon. She thought I looked dreadful and after hearing my story suggested that I visit Leonie who did wonders with necks and backs. I had nothing to lose, so I dragged myself slowly up the stairs that same day; and so began a course of treatment which has helped me in so many ways.

Medical practitioners who understood — at last

Leonie's many years of experience and tremendous presence, inspire confidence in those around her. She initially began her training in physiotherapy, eventually turning to chiropractic, osteopathy, acupuncture and homoeopathy. Osteopathy is her specialty and it is such a gentle practice that it is very suitable for the wretched joints and muscles of those 'tied up in knots' with ME/CFS. (Osteopathy is the gentle art of manipulation of soft tissue, such as fascia, ligaments and muscles. It is often used in conjunction with chiropractic manipulations. To demonstrate the difference — the philosophy of osteopathy is 'The Rule of the Artery is Supreme' whereas the philosophy of chiropractic is 'Structure governs Function'.) Leonie has an amazing amount of practical information and home remedies, some of which I have mentioned later in this book.

I quickly realised that I had not only found an expert in her field, but a true friend. She did not treat me as a neurotic woman, but discovered that I had four ribs out of place. She massaged me and then gently lifted me off my feet. The relief was enormous. She did not tell me until a couple of years later that my body was in a dangerous state of stress, that my muscles had lost their elasticity and that she expected me to end up in a wheelchair. I told her I was booked in to see Dr Eric and she said he was extremely clever and that it was an excellent course to follow.

Dr Eric darted into the waiting room and escorted me into his surgery. I took to him immediately as I wended my way through the array of children's toys to a chair. He is one of the most interesting people I have ever met. He is natural, unpretentious and appears to have a photographic memory. His mind is ticking over all the time you are there — he does not miss a thing. And he gave me *time*.

After I had explained the history of my illness, he asked me the most unusual questions — 'Do you feel angry? Is it sore on the right side or the left side? Do you feel cold or heat? Are you thirsty? Do you want to be cuddled or left alone?' (These questions, I subsequently discovered, were based on homoepathic methods of treatment, discussed in a later chapter.) He did the usual checks with the stethoscope, looked through all my previous blood tests and then took a small torch and looked into my eyes. He mentioned something about the lymphatics and the liver and said, 'I think you have Myalgic Encephalomyelitis'. This did not mean a thing to me at the time, but at least he seemed to *know* what was wrong with me. He took some blood to be sent away for analysis and said it would take time to recover. I was to start some medicines he called 'remedies' which were dispensed at his surgery. They did look a little strange, but I thought I had nothing to lose and Aunty Hay, my friend in her eighties, had said they worked wonders.

So I began a course of treatment which has proved incredibly effective for me. One of the remedies produced a most unexpected result. I became so angry for about ten days that my husband wondered what was wrong with me. (This was followed by a feeling of great calmness.) I mentioned this to Dr Eric who just laughed and said, 'that was to bring out your anger'. It was during this course of treatment that my daughter was married and the reception for 84 people was held at our home. There was a great deal to be done as, with the help of friends, we organised it ourselves. However it all went off smoothly thanks to the gradual improvement in my state of health.

Leonie encouraged me to read as much as I could about homoeopathy. She lent me many books so that I could understand how I was being treated. As I seemed to be faced with a fairly long-term illness, I figured I had to take responsibility for my illness and do as much as I could to help myself. Being of a very determined nature I was not going to give in without a very hard battle, so it seemed logical that I try to understand my treatment.

I did indeed make very good progress during those six months of treatment with Dr Eric and Leonie. Dr Eric was strongly supportive of Leonie's approach and would often send me back to her for treatment. (I found this situation most unusual — a doctor actually recommending the services of a chiropractor/osteopath). During weekly visits to Leonie I continued my massage, lymphatic drainage (which is encouraged by massage) and acupuncture treatment to calm the nervous system, and saw Dr Eric about once a month. By late July I was feeling much more like my old self again and, as my husband was a very enthusiastic skier, I agreed to go with him once again.

Not realising the jeopardy in which I was placing myself we returned to the same ski lodge with the same dreadful smell. I skied for one afternoon, had to drag myself back up the steps to the ski lodge, and within two days I had such difficulty breathing and felt so ill we had to come home.

First relapse, August 1984

I was back in bed again with a severe relapse. Dr Eric came to the rescue with more remedies and a course of homoeopathic injections made from a few drops of my own blood which made me feel on top of the world. However, because I thought I was cured I accelerated my lifestyle once again, exposed myself to toxic chemicals, had a couple of further minor relapses, took more remedies and finally I went away for a holiday on the mid-north coast in January 1985.

After the break I improved immensely and it was about this time that Leonie danced around the massage table when she saw that my body had returned to normal. My muscles were working and had regained their elasticity. She said I had to thank Dr Eric for my life because he had drained me of toxins. I might add here that Dr Eric insists that I have Leonie to thank, also, as many times he referred me back to her for acupuncture and other treatment. He is one of the few doctors who recognise the worth of osteopathic, acupuncture and chiropractic treatment. If branches of the medical profession would work more closely together incorporating these ancillary practitioners, and would consider the whole person rather than just one aspect or symptom of their illness, the patient would be the beneficiary (e.g. a heap of pills taken for back pain will only relieve the pain, they will not cure the *cause* of the problem.)

During the course of my treatment I was introduced by Dr Eric to a couple of marvellous herbal remedies. The first,

Echinacea, has the most remarkable effect. It tones up the body, builds up the immune system and gives you energy; that is not only my experience but also that of various members of my family and a couple of friends. The other is Chelidonium, which Dr Eric incorporates into a liver drainage programme. These two remedies had a very dramatic effect on my healing processes.

At this time, February 1985, I was extremely well, except for a slight digestive problem. Being a perfectionist I wanted to be 100 per cent well, and as there was a tummy parasite prevalent at the time, Dr Eric thought this may be the cause. He put me on Flagyl (anti-parasitic). The taste and smell of this was horrible and I could barely get it down. I developed severe thrush (candida) again and started gradually sliding downhill.

Second relapse

In March, while visiting friends in the country, I endured three hours of exposure to dichlorvos and heptachlor which were being sprayed in the house while we were standing on the verandah. The smell absolutely repulsed me at the time. Later in the day, my eyes streamed and my arms and legs burned. Over a period of two weeks I gradually got weaker and weaker until, after spending a night with cigarette smokers in a small room, I relapsed into the worst ME/CFS symptoms I could ever describe. My body was like lead and I felt I was sinking through the mattress. My body burned under the skin yet was freezing cold, I could not keep my eyelids up, could not eat, could hardly speak and I had to concentrate on breathing. Every time I moved a muscle my whole body shuddered and vibrated. It was even more terrifying than the previous relapse. I felt so desperately ill I thought I was dying.

Dr Eric had been treating me with homoeopathic Kali Carb just prior to my collapse and he, unfortunately for me, was now away on four weeks holiday.

The GP standing in for him was not familiar with my case. He gave me the same injections I had had previously but this time they did not work. I was just too sick to trail around, I could not walk and my husband almost had to carry me everywhere. Leonie visited me at home and was shocked at the deterioration of my muscles. I really thought that this time I would die for sure! I was not frightened but felt so ill that I did not care what happened to me. I remember ringing my daughter to say I may not make it through the night. My weight had dropped to 39kg (6 stone 2 lbs).

My husband has reminded me of a conversation we had during this time of extreme illness when I had been bedridden for some time — it was the middle of winter and extremely cold.

'Hello, darling, I'm home. Would you like me to cook some brains in parsley sauce for tea? I bought them especially for you.'

'No, Paul, I have been thinking. I have been such a nuisance to you and the whole family, you would certainly be able to find a much better wife than I've turned out to be, so I am going to go out into the cold, catch pneumonia, die, and then you won't have to worry about me any more.'

'Does that mean you don't want brains?'

'No, I don't.'

Door opens and closes. Five minutes pass. Door opens.

'I see you're back again. Not going to end it all?'

'No, it was too cold out there.'

'Would you like some brains then?'

'Yes, please, I'll try to eat a little.'

We have laughed about this since, but possibly you have felt this way too, for it is a long, long haul back to some sort of normality. You won't die from ME/CFS, you'll just wish you could!

Finally Dr Eric returned from holidays, my husband literally carried me to him and with two or three doses of homoeopathic Nux Vomica I started to feel better. It is obviously very important to have a good and trusting relationship with your medical practitioner. I was not leaping around by any stretch of the imagination, but I was able to get out of bed to make an urgent trip to the mid-north coast of New South Wales in order to sign the contract to build our holiday cottage.

Although I began to improve slowly I also had another series of relapses which, in retrospect, I realise were brought on by exposure to cigarette smoke, cleaning products, fly spray and disinfectant. Then I developed two abscessed teeth. The elderly dentist I had attended for years was at a loss to know what to do as Dr Eric had said to avoid antibiotics. He drained the worst tooth, and then put chloro-phenol into the tooth. The taste and smell revolted me. I could not wait to get home to wash it out. Within several hours I developed the burning under the skin again and went into severe relapse. Dr Eric realised at this point that I was acutely sensitive to petrochemicals and maybe formaldehyde.

It was as though he had found the key to the locked door. As we went back through my case history, we realised that every relapse had been brought on by exposure to toxic chemicals including drugs, and the pesticides had been the worst of all. I had not thought to tell Dr Eric that I had been exposed to them because I did not know just how dangerous they could be.

My tooth problem was solved with the homoeopathic remedies Pyrogen and Staph, I found a new and open-minded dentist, the abscess cleared up and I have been able to keep both molars without recourse to antibiotics.

It was a long haul back to health after this relapse which was followed by a series of further relapses. I followed the same treatment pattern as before with homoeopathic and herbal remedies coupled with Leonie's marvellous therapy. This time I really concentrated on cleaning up my environment so as to avoid relapse.

It was obvious that my home was contributing to my illness. It had polished floors and stairs, oil heating and was situated alongside a golf course which was subject to various chemical sprays and treatments. We lived in a hollow where the pollution settled. But I loved the house. It was very large, split-level, an architect's dream home and my first husband and I had built it with our bare hands. I had put so much hard work into it and landscaped most of the garden. It was the first home I had ever owned and the thought of selling tore me apart. At this stage I was far from well. My strength would disappear at the slightest exertion and I had to resort to getting help with the housework — something I considered a terrible extravagance. However, one had to be logical. If I did not sell up and make a move to a more practical home, away from pollution, I might never get better.

My husband loved our home also. Since moving in on the day we were married, he had contributed in no small way to finishing off all the jobs which had been left undone. He was not at all enthusiastic at the thought of leaving but, bless him, he did realise we had no option if I was to concentrate on regaining my health.

At the end of January 1986 I had to make a move. I glanced through the paper and saw a house advertised which sounded suitable. I put my own house on the market. Looking at houses when one is feeling as weak as a kitten is not really the best thing to do, but it had to be done. So, insisting that the real estate agents transport me to and fro, off I went. Unbelievably, the first house I looked at had everything that I needed, even the bonus of a non-chemical swimming pool and it was on the edge of a national park away from pollution. What more could I ask? I figured it must be God's will as I sold my own home within three days of it being advertised.

The move did not all go smoothly, however. There were complications in selling my house, my daughter was very unhappy about the move and Paul's commitments at work had increased. Although a country friend helped considerably, on some days my strength would disappear altogether.

Sometimes I wonder how we managed it but in April I found myself sitting on the verandah of my new abode, surrounded by packing cases. Paul was a tower of strength during the actual move.

I had learned to be sensible and established the new household only very gradually over a period of many weeks. I spent a great deal of time sitting outside looking at the garden and planning just how I would change it to suit both my personality and that of the house, which was very Australian in character and needed a bush setting. Some days I would walk down to the letterbox and wonder how my legs would carry me back.

As the weeks went by I gradually began to improve. I had thrown out all the products containing toxic chemicals which I had previously used, found new safe alternatives, and found myself a house on the top of a hill, as far from pollution as possible. It worked! For two years I did not suffer a relapse but it did take all that time to regain my strength.

These were wonderful days. I felt great. My daughter had produced her first child. I had the garden looking lovely, having re-landscaped it myself with the help of my husband who pushed the heavy barrow. I now had a lovely solar-heated swimming pool which used, instead of chemicals, an ionic exchange purification system (see directory, page 221). We had some renovations done and my health did not deteriorate as I was careful to avoid any noxious fumes. I was ready and able to enjoy life and finally the little cottage we had built on the mid-north coast had lost most of its toxicity. I was able to stay there without problems. The paints, glues, varnishes and carpet were the worst offenders as it takes a long time for the fumes to 'blow out'.

I explained my problems to all the neighbours. It took a little time for them to understand, but they have been wonderfully cooperative and have changed their own attitudes to dangerous chemicals as a result. Paul and I established a lovely bush garden around our holiday home and life was really wonderful.

At this stage Echinacea was a marvellous tonic. I had changed my diet to control and clear up my thrush (discussed fully later) and although I was now eating no bread or yeast at all, I put on over 6kg in weight. My health was so good once again that I was not tired and I was sleeping at night.

In March 1988 I minded my 11 months old granddaughter for five days and coped marvellously. So much so that when my daughter returned to collect her I did not want to part with her. It was the morning of 25 March. I shall not forget the day as Paul and I had planned to leave that afternoon to spend a few days at our holiday cottage. I was standing by the edge of the swimmng pool giving it a last clean-up when I noticed a strange smell waft over my property carried on a north-east breeze. It did not have a petrochemical base (I get a sore throat and nose immediately) but it made my eyes hurt. As it was not any smell I was familiar with, and as it seemed to pass away within 20 minutes or so, I did not worry too much about it but went on with my preparations to leave in the mid-afternoon. As we drove along I started to become very agitated and worried about the drive (something I never do as Paul is a wonderful driver), eventually becoming quite hysterical and feeling most unwell. By the time we arrived at our cottage I could barely drag myself into the house, make the bed and collapse into it.

Third relapse

By the next morning I had all the old symptoms — nausea, swollen glands, body pains like acute arthritis and rheumatism in every joint and muscle. All I wanted was boiled water to drink and I ate nothing for three days. I lost 3.5 kg. I spent the holiday unable to do anything.

As soon as we returned to Sydney I went to see Dr Eric. Typical ME/CFS relapse was his diagnosis. Upon our return home we noticed the dead grass in the adjoining street and in a direct line north-east from where I had been standing alongside the pool when I encountered the strange smell. I rang the Council and discovered they *had* sprayed in March with the herbicide Amitrole without letting me know, (although I had a letter from them saying that they would always let me know if they were spraying in my area), but they would not admit to spraying on that particular day. I spoke to all the neighbours in that area but no-one had had any spraying done. I can only deduce it was the herbicide, but have no proof.

It is really worrying to be so chemically sensitive and know that you can be knocked down with such ease as it takes a long time to get back up again. It makes a healthy life very tenuous!

Although this last relapse was nowhere near as bad as the previous ones, it took me the best part of nine months to get my strength back.

I notice that with each successive exposure and relapse I have become more chemically sensitive and have developed other symptoms I did not previously have. I must state here that it sometimes takes a day or two for an exposure to take effect; it is not always instantaneous, which makes it more difficult to pinpoint the culprit. Also, excessive exertion does not always bring on immediate fatigue — this can take some hours to develop. ME/CFS is a strange malady!

In February 1989 I went trout fishing and was able to walk miles, but while there I contracted a cold with flu-like symptoms. I was fortunate that I needed only one day in bed when the aches were bad and I had a 'wonderful' temperature of 101 degrees — it delighted me as I knew that my immune system was working again.

So here I am sharing my experiences with you and offering hope of a more fulfilling and healthy life in the future. It will take '*the capacity to affect great changes*' in our attitudes, our home and work environment and our approach to medicine. Nevertheless when we begin the changes our minds are opened to nature and all that stems from Creation. I hope you find the following pages interesting and helpful.

<h1>3   The Immune System</h1>

As ME/CFS seems to be a malfunction or deficiency of the immune system it is essential to avoid the things which depress the immune system and to devote oneself to building it up. One of the purposes of this book is to alert everyone to the potential hazards to our immune system and general health and to suggest remedies and therapies which will strengthen it. That is the key to recovery from ME/CFS.

I attended a seminar on ME in Sydney two years ago which was held by the Australian Medical Faculty of Homoeopathy. The guest speaker was Professor Wakefield. He, as stated previously, is concerned with research currently being undertaken into this bizarre disease. During his lecture he stated 'We know what puts the immune system *down*, but we don't know enough about what *builds it up*'. Since then, although a great deal has been learned about the workings of the immune system, we are still looking for a complete cure.

I had the opportunity to address this particular seminar, being the only ME/CFS patient there. Dr Eric and I had prepared and sent our questionnaire (see page 201) to many of his patients and the results had come back with overwhelming evidence of chemical sensitivity. This he tendered at the conference. Other than the questionnaire results, the question of chemical toxicity was not discussed until I raised it at the end of the proceedings. Unfortunately

Professor Wakefield had departed. However, I did ask those present to consider the possibility that ME/CFS could be the result of exposure to, or overload of, noxious chemicals. I wonder whether any of them ever gave this question consideration?

What Puts the Immune System 'Down'?

- a severe virus or infection will debilitate the immune system.
- innoculations and vaccinations, by altering the balance of 'T' cells.
- antibiotics, by destroying healthy bacteria.
- other drugs, including steroids (eg cortisone), the contraceptive pill, cancer chemotherapy, interferon, and many other medications. Many toxic chemicals are used in the manufacture of pharmaceuticals including pesticide, phenol, formaldehyde, chloroform and perchloroethylene. These can depress the immune system and/or affect the nervous system. Perfect examples are the preparations sold for the treatment of head lice which contain maldison or lindane.

  (*Lindane* is an organochlorine and, besides causing nervous system damage, is highly suspected of causing cancer. Organochlorines may be stored in the body fat for a long period. *Maldison* is an organophosphate. Organophosphates will inactivate cholinesterase enzymes which are essential to the function of the nervous system. *Phenol* is used in the production of aspirin and other drugs.)
- transfusion reactions.
- stress, including feelings of resentment, hatred, guilt, envy, anger and greed, particularly if it is continuous.
- overtiredness.

- chilling: how often have you heard the advice 'Don't stand in a cold draft or you will catch a cold'? This has been dismissed as an 'old wives' tale' but when the body is chilled it does seem to have an adverse effect on the immune system, making us more susceptible to viruses or bacteria.
- toxic chemicals, including some pesticides, herbicides, petrochemicals, formaldehyde and solvents. (For further information see the chapter 'Pesticides, Herbicides and Other Toxic Chemicals'.)

What Builds up the Immune System?
- gamma-globulin serum and transfer factor (by infusion and injection).
- relaxation, meditation, rest and prayer.
- vitamins and/or minerals if you have a deficiency.
- herbal remedies: Echinacea and Phytolacca which have a beneficial effect on the blood count and Chelidonium which assists in clearing the liver of toxins.
- homoeopathic vaccines/medicines.
- eating a balanced diet of naturally grown uncontaminated foods and living in a relaxed, non-toxic environment.

As you can see there are many factors in our daily environment which adversely affect our immune system, and not very many which help to build it up unless we make the effort ourselves.

One of the greatest problems we face today is the 'quick fix' mentality. When we get a cold or flu we expect the doctor to hand us a prescription for an instant cure, instead of taking the rest which is necessary for the immune system to muster its forces and thus cure us. We should be working with nature instead of against it, otherwise we will fail in the long run. We do not stop to think that it is our own immune system which will ultimately affect the cure. We pop our pills and keep on working, making the job so much more difficult for the natural healing processes to take place. We should be doing everything possible to help the immune response as suggested in this chapter and rest is essential in times of sickness.

II Understanding the triggers

4   Pesticides, Herbicides and Other Toxic Chemicals

Some of the known harmful effects

It was not until I became ill and realised the effects that toxic chemicals were having on my own health that I became interested in this subject at all — such is the way of most of us. In most cases unless we, or someone close to us, are personally affected, we do not start to think seriously about our health and environment. We tend to shrug it off and think 'that will not happen to me'. I hope that people who read this book, but do not believe that they are personally being affected, will start to realise that they *are* being affected by the toxic pollution all around us. Here are some facts in brief as supplied by Dr Kate Short from the Total Environment Centre, Sydney:

> Pesticides and many other toxic chemicals are not tested as to their effects on the immune system before marketing. Organochlorine pesticides accumulate in the body, poison the liver, are linked to cancer, affect the immune system and the production of hormones. Aldrin, dieldrin, chlordane and heptachlor, all organochlorines, have been withdrawn or restricted in the majority of western countries including USA and many organophosphate and

carbamate pesticides are much more restricted in their use in other developed countries.

Dr Ian Nisbet, Consultant Toxicologist from Boston, Massachusetts and a world authority on organochlorines was interviewed at length regarding aldrin, dieldrin, chlordane and heptachlor on 'Earthworm' ABC radio during March 1989. His findings, after reviewing all relevant studies, many of which were unpublished, show that chlordane and heptachlor cause cancer in mice and rats and possibly in humans. Although chlordane is the most hazardous, none of the other organochlorines can be regarded as safe as they also cause adverse effects on the liver and kidneys, adverse reproductive effects and affect the immune system. The exact doses at which these occur and the exact exposures differ from chemical to chemical. *All are no longer used in the USA and have been successfully replaced by safer, effective alternatives*, according to Dr Nisbet.

The studies on animals exposed to components of chlordane show that it affects the immune system at very low levels of exposure. Immune effects in humans can vary — exposure might produce colds, chemical sensitisation, stomach-aches, nausea, headaches, or no effect at all. Study of the immune system is a developing field of science and the effects on the immune system may be one of the most serious problems that exposure to chemicals in the environment is causing in the population. Many toxicologists believe we are only seeing the tip of the iceberg and Dr Nisbet subscribes to this view. The effects of chlordane and heptachlor on the reproductive system of rabbits and rats at very low levels of exposure is disturbing and Dr Nisbet wonders why this material has been overlooked by many health authorities.

Most of the studies commissioned by the manufacturers have not been available to the general public. Dr Nisbet has reviewed fourteen such studies. Some conclusions given to the manufacturers did not reflect the contained data in the studies. At one point the US Environmental

Protection Agency began criminal proceedings against the manufacturers of chlordane for failure to report adverse findings of cancer studies in mice. Not only did the studies reveal that these pesticides can cause cancer but also that they had other detrimental effects on the liver, kidneys, immune system, nervous system and reproductive system. The EPA was so caught up in the cancer issue that the other toxic effects have been ignored by them, Dr Nisbet said.

According to Dr Nisbet one reason why these pesiticides may not have been banned in all countries is that other scientists have not had access to those studies (which were commissioned by the manufacturers), and have not really reviewed the data adequately.

Chlordane and heptachlor are on the list of suspected carcinogens as supplied by the New South Wales Division of Occupational Health. However both are still permitted for use sub-soil for termites in New South Wales.

The more I investigated the effects of toxic chemicals, and the more information I received regarding pesticides, the more alarmed I became. It is just amazing that everyone has been so complacent about it. It is only now, because our environment is threatened and export products are in jeopardy from pesticide residues, that the government is really beginning to take some notice.

Certainly the media has taken up the issue recently because, with the strange weather we have been experiencing, the talk of Greenhouse effect and ozone levels, sewage and residue problems, people are becoming much more aware! Hardly a week goes by when we don't hear about a toxic chemical fire or spill somewhere. People have to be evacuated and there is danger of pollution.

The Toxic and Hazardous Chemicals Committee of the Total Environment Centre undertook a study entitled 'A Multidisciplinary Analysis of Pesticide Related Problems in New South Wales' by Robert H.J. Verkerk B.Sc (Hons.). The report, dated January 1987, is available from the Centre (see directory) and contains some very worrying information. With permission, I am setting down some extracts from the report.

> In 1975 the Department of Agriculture conducted staff briefings in each region on the matter of organo-chlorine residues and methods of avoiding them. Ironically the North Coast Regional Seminar was conducted in Kempsey itself, on June 3rd 1975. The Department of Agriculture has been quarantining farms since 1976 due to excessive heptachlor and dieldrin residues. Despite this, farmers in the Coffs Harbour, Bellingen, Nambucca, Macleay, Hastings and Manning Shires received written recommendations for the use of heptachlor on dairy farms for Spring 1977/Summer 1978. These must have been given with the full knowledge of the problems and implications.

> It may be assumed that in most cases up to fifteen years are required for organo-chlorine pesticides to break down sufficiently so that residues in grazing stock will not exceed the MRLs (maximum residue levels). If the Department of Agriculture had heeded warnings in the early to mid 1970s and banned the agricultural uses of these products at that time, in line with the United States, the residues would not have been allowed to accumulate to their present critical state. The cost of this delay must now be borne in terms of both analysis and management of the residue problem.

> The nine year delay between the Department of Agriculture's full knowledge of the implications of continuing the use of organo-chlorines (1975) and their effective withdrawal from the dairy industry (1984) appears to have been politically motivated and irresponsible since it neglected to support the most efficient production of food. The same applies to the deliberate withholding of information from dairy farmers from the 30th October

1981 (the effective promulgation of the Pesticides Act, 1978) to the 22nd May 1984, the date of the Minister for Agriculture's press release on the subject. The Department maintains that these decisions were made for fear of adverse publicity of residues in milk by local environmental groups.

We will take a break from the report whilst still on the subject of milk. In 1987 there was a scare on the mid-north coast regarding the levels of dieldrin in the milk due to the animals being fed on a dieldrin-treated grain feed mix. My husband, who lived in the country in the 1960s, tells me on some farms it was recognised practice to wash the wheat in dieldrin before it was placed in the silos. (According to a farmer I know this practice is still used on some properties, although other pesticides, including organophosphates are now used instead of organochlorines.) My husband mixed the dieldrin with his bare hands. I have been informed by a spokesman from the NSW Division of Occupational Health that silos were treated with organochlorines before the wheat was stored and that those storage areas are being phased out. (Organochlorines are no longer permitted in the wheat industry.)

Now back to the report:

Very briefly, the four known mechanisms of toxicity for organo-chlorine insecticides are:

1 neurotoxicity: competitive inhibition of one specific enzyme in brain-specific sites (Beeman and Matsumura, 1981).

2 membrane damage, due to accumulation in the lipid phase of membranes as a result of high lipid solubility. Those membranes involved in cellular respiration are particularly affected.

3 potential for free-radical formation and DNA damage; highly reactive free-radicals may be formed. These free-radicals and their reaction products may damage DNA, causing delayed effect such as mutagenesis (Nakayama et al., 1984; Reynolds and Moslew, 1980).

4 *immune system dysregulation and chemical sensitivity; the mechanisms are poorly understood, but they cause the sufferer to become ultra-sensitive to specific groups of chemicals.* (Author's emphasis)

A final point concerns the significance of MRLs in regard to human health. An extract from a Department of Agriculture publication 'Pesticide Residues and the Stock Owner' (*Agfact* AO. 9.30, second edition, 1984) reads:

Feeding studies on laboratory animals are used to establish the level at which no effect is shown in the most susceptible species. These no-effect residue levels are then reduced to provide a large safety factor (normally 100 times) to calculate the MRL. Thus the NHMRC (National Health and Medical Research Council) MRL is well below the level toxic to humans.

This interpretation has severe limitations:

1 With lipid soluble compounds like organo-chlorines, which tend to accumulate, differences in exposure of individuals becomes highly relevant.

2 Related compounds which exert a similar and cumulative effect are not taken into account in the MRL, such as organo-chlorines of non-pesticide origins, e.g. poly-chlorinated byphenyls, tetrachloroethylene etc., which are relatively more abundant.

3 Differences in genetic susceptibility. By virtue of the heterogeneous nature of the human genotype, certain individuals are considerably more susceptible

to the effects of chemicals than others. This contrasts sharply with the homogeneous genetic make-up of the laboratory animals from which the MRLs are derived.

The Department of Agriculture has apparently shown no significant interest in the activities of biodynamic farmers, David and Helen Williams, who cultivate wheat and rye on approximately 300 acres of the more marginal lands in the Breeza Plains. Biodynamic farming techniques do not involve the use of chemical fertilisers or pesticides, instead relying on a long term rotation for weed control and nutrient build-up. Specially prepared microbiological (biodynamic) sprays are applied to increase vigour of crop plants and legumes may be planted to increase nitrogen levels, whilst livestock may be allowed to graze to assist in natural fertilisation. Productivity on this farm is between 0.75t(onne) and 1.2t/acre and is generally greater than that of conventional farms in the drier years. This wheat commands a premium price on the world market.

Included in this pesticide report from which the above information is quoted were a number of case histories. The report also states that in 1981 more than 500 people in Gunnedah were diagnosed as suffering from ME/CFS. Dr David Cook, a local GP was affected, too. He suspected that the sprays from the cotton growers which drifted over the area were in some way involved as patients worsened during such times. Dr Cook tells me that there are still many sick people in Gunnedah and more cases of ME/CFS have been diagnosed.

I know a couple in Gunnedah who own a lovely property in the area but are afraid to build on it because of the close proximity of cotton fields and the consequent frequent spraying. My friend suffers from asthma. The land has been owned by the family for many, many years long before cotton was grown in the area. Needless to say they are angry and disappointed.

There are also a number of ME/CFS cases cited in the report which developed after pest treatments in their own homes or on the adjoining property. I somehow feel that ME/CFS victims will be treated much as the Vietnam veterans who are still trying to prove their case against the manufacturers of Agent Orange, yet they know in their own minds and bodies why they are ill.

Toxic chemicals are absorbed in three ways:

1 by inhalation: 'Our lungs have the capacity of a sponge the size of a tennis court' (*Chemical Victims* — Dr Mackarness).
2 by ingestion via the food and drink we put into our mouth.
3 absorption through the skin and eyes.

Unfortunately we can be exposed to pesticides and other toxins without our knowledge, especially in the case of residual sprays which can be picked up on the hands and from vaporisation, etc. This can occur in the workplace as regular treatments are given to office, shop and factory buildings. We can catch the drift in the air from a pesticide or herbicide treatment some hundreds of metres away from where we happen to be, as happened to me last year. It is also possible for aerial spray drifts to travel hundreds of kilometres under high wind conditions.

In October 1987 I was most unwell for no apparent reason and I was puzzled. My friends with ME/CFS were sick too. The air was very dry because of the south-westerly winds blowing and I was constantly plagued by the unpleasant effect the outside air was having on my nose and throat. I felt continuously fatigued and I could find no good reason.

I telephoned the Department of Agriculture and spoke to a senior official to see if any aerial spraying was taking place as I had heard that there was the beginning of a locust plague in the west and south-west of New South

Wales. Perhaps this could account for my malaise. I was told that climatic conditions had not necessitated the spraying of locusts because the cold weather had taken care of them.

A few weeks later, by sheer accident, I saw a copy of *The Land* (15 October 1987) which stated that 'large scale aerial spraying with organophosphorus insecticide' had taken place in the south-west and west of the State for over a week. Maybe the Pastures Protection Board and Department of Agriculture do not communicate.

Besides aerial 'drift' of sprays we can be exposed in our homes or workplace. It is interesting to note that Baygon, a well-known household surface spray, which contained dichlorvos, an organophosphate, now contains only propoxur a carbamate. Carbamates and organophospates are inhibitors of cholinesterase (an essential enzyme of the central nervous system). Although carbamates are allegedly not as dangerous as organophosphates they rate three out of three on the scale of toxicity as supplied by the Division of Occupational Health (see pages 53, 54).

The dangers of dichlorvos were brought to the notice of the public in the *Sun-Herald* (20 December, 1987) by Senator Coulter, a research scientist by profession. He told the Senate that 'tests in 1973 had shown dichlorvos was a mutagen and in the US *Chemical Regulation Reporter* of 7 July 1987 a National Toxicology Program advisory panel on July 14 approved a draft report concluding that the pesticide clearly caused cancer in male rats and female mice.'

An inquiry to Nicholas Kiwi Pty Ltd, now the marketers of Shelltox Pest Strips and dog and cat flea bands, revealed the following:

> Mini Pest Strips 186 grams per kilogram dichlorvos
> Maxi Pest Strips 192 grams per kilogram dichlorvos
> Dog Bands 97 grams per kilogram dichlorvos
> Cat Bands 30 grams per kilogram dichlorvos
> They carry the warning 'ANTI-CHOLINESTERASE'.

I am making an example of these products which have been so freely advertised and sold in the stores. To their credit Bayer have removed dichlorvos from Baygon.

Dichlorvos has been used by pest controllers for house and office fumigation. It is registered for a wide variety of household pests. The acute effects of the chemical include flu-like symptoms, muscle twitching and paralysis. It can also cause allergic skin reaction, breathing difficulties and precipitate severe asthma attacks.

Exposure to dichlorvos has in the opinion of both myself and a number of others, contributed to our severe relapses into the ME/CFS syndrome.

I have a young acquaintance who at the age of twelve was exposed to dichlorvos when her mother used a surface spray containing this pesticide in her kitchen. My young friend collapsed and was rushed to hospital where she eventually recovered. However, her health gradually deteriorated with throat and other infections which eventually led to throat surgery. When her schooling was finally completed she was advised not to take a job or undertake a course of study as her health was so poor — she needed at least a year's rest. Unfortunately, during this period she visited a friend and was once again exposed to dichlorvos which she believes put her into severe ME/CFS relapse from which she has never recovered. That was five years ago. She is at last making some headway with the gamma-globulin and transfer factor coupled with alternative therapies. However, she is still severely invalided, extremely chemically sensitive, spends most of her time resting in bed and has great difficulty speaking. What a tragedy for such a young person.

You will remember my mention of some head lice preparations in my chapter on 'The Immume system'. The local chemist was quite horrified when I told her of the possible effects of both lindane and maldison. There is no warning on the packaging that they may cause cancer and/or nervous system damage, only that they are to be used with caution. This would seem to be worrying when the growing incidence of cancer and leukaemia in children is of great concern to everyone.

I was listening to 'Body Talk' on Radio 2GB Sydney one Saturday evening when a very eminent doctor, who was doing research into genetic engineering at the Children's Hospital in Sydney, was being interviewed. He said the incidence of cancer and leukemia in small children was of great concern and they were finding that 'good genes' which fight cancer were being 'shut down'. The reason for this was a mystery. I telephoned him and asked whether he had considered the possibility of this 'shut down' being caused by toxic chemicals, particularly pesticides. His reply was, 'That is very intuitive of you. We are looking at that possibility, however it is a very difficult area of research'. The possible ramifications of all this are not pleasant to contemplate.

According to the New South Wales Department of Agriculture, the following chemicals are registered for termite control in buildings:
- aldrin, dieldrin, chlordane heptachlor (organochlorines)
- chlorpyrifos (organophosphate)
- arsenic trioxide

All are extremely poisonous and, at least until 1989, no other treatments or chemicals are registered.

There are safer alternatives being used overseas including pyrethroids which are registered only for cockroaches and other household and agricultural pests at present. There is no doubt there should be far more education of people generally regarding the potential health hazards of many pesticides and far more emphasis on chemical free, safe alternatives.

Chlordane was eventually restricted in New South Wales in January 1987. However it could still be purchased from a country hardware store in 1988 and was sold to a neighbour of mine for black ant control. He had no idea of the toxicity of this organochlorine pesticide or that it had been withdrawn from sale to the general public. Chlordane is only permitted for use subsoil for termites (white ants) and cannot be sold over the counter.

There is no need to use the above pesticides. There are safe alternatives. We have built a holiday house where there is a real termite problem. The house was built on brick piers with lead flashing so that it is easy to observe any termite workings. The pest controller makes two inspections per year. We have not used toxic chemicals. Upon inquiry from various councils both in the city and country I have discovered that if building or extending it is not necessarily compulsory to have the building site treated for termites. For example, the Kuring-gai Council, Sydney, does not require such a treatment. However the Hastings Municipal Council, does.

In the Blue Mountains of New South Wales where termite treatment of new constructions is regulatory, more than fifty doctors signed a petition calling for a ban on the use of organochlorine pesticides claiming they cause cancer. At a council meeting in December 1988 Dr John England, a heart specialist, called on aldermen to 'put people first — not the legalities of the law'. Council aldermen are concerned by the fact that the Environmental Protection Agency in the USA has had the pesticides withdrawn because they are neurotoxic, bio-accumulative, cause infertility and are toxic to bone marrow, especially in children. Alderman Scott Whitehair said he was prepared to break the law by banning the 'carcinogenic' sprays and if Council was to be sued he would rather it be by people suffering from termites than cancer. Alderman Lawton told council that the intent of the law was to stop people's homes being eaten by termites, not to expose them to carcinogenic chemicals.

It was finally resolved by council that provided the owner of the property notified the council in writing that he/she took full responsibility for any subsequent termite (white ant) damage, the council would not require the use of toxic chemicals for the treatment of termites.

Just when I thought I had educated my surrounding

neighbours, once again we had to return to Sydney from our holiday cottage because of pest treatments. In September 1989 the owner of the land opposite us decided to commence building. His land consists of a sand dune fronting the ocean. The bitou bush and dune wattle were bulldozed off and the sand levelled so that a concrete slab could be poured upon which the house was to be constructed. The Hastings Municipal Council requires as a condition of the granting of a building permit that 'the area beneath concrete floor to be treated to prevent termite attack and a certificate from a recognised firm of pest exterminators prepared in accordance with AS/2057/1989 is to be produced to council to verify same prior to the pouring of the slab'. Inquiries from Systems Pest Management Services Pty Ltd in Sydney advised that applying the registered chemicals, namely chlordane, heptachlor, aldrin and dieldrin or chlorpyrifos (organophosphate) would not be effective in sand, particularly almost white sand, as there is virtually no organic material to bind with the chemical selected and it would leach straight into the ocean.

The matter was taken up with the Building Inspector who said that he was bound by the regulations but if the owner chose to take full responsibility for subsequent termite infestation and submitted a letter to the effect that he was not having the sand sprayed for environmental reasons, the Council would give the required permit. According to the Building Inspector, if the council approved a building without any form of termite prevention then they would be liable. If an infestation occurs within the time of limitation of the pest controller's certificate then he is responsible. My new neighbour, who is a very nice and reasonable man, saw the virtual uselessness of such treatment. However, after discussion with Council, he was not prepared to take the responsibility and as there was no safe alternative treatment registered for termite control, he decided to have the sand dune sprayed.

Our holiday was shortened by one week. Our roof had to be washed thoroughly and the water tank drained so that any drift from the treatment did not contaminate our drinking water.

Obviously the fact that much of our coastal development is either on sand or light sandy soil has not been a consideration when the registration of chemicals for termite control originally took place.

The *Sydney Morning Herald* of 9 September 1989 reports

samples of fish caught in the Newcastle area of New South Wales have revealed pesticide levels nearly five times higher than the limits recommended by the National Health and Medical Research Council.

According to the results of the samples, locally caught morwong and groper respectively contained chlordane levels 4.6 times and 5.3 times higher than the maximum limits under NHMRC guidelines.

He [Mr Moore, the NSW Minister for Environment] said that of the 12 pesticides tested for, only chlordane was found in amounts exceeding health limits and that these were lower than those found in fish caught around sewage outfalls in and around Sydney. (Samples of fish recently caught around Malabar outfall revealed chlordane/oxychlordane levels approximately 12 times higher than the recommended health levels).

However, another pesticide, heptachlor and heptachlor epoxide — commonly used in site preparations for the control of termites — were also detected in fish at approximately half the maximum limit set by the NHMRC.

All the other pesticides were found in minute amounts, well below the recommended levels, he said.

The report is disturbing as it indicates that, as in Sydney, pesticides are entering the ocean apparently through sewage and urban runoff (my emphasis).

According to the article, further testing is to take place and the Hunter Water Board has recently released a new trade waste policy with significantly tightened discharge limits and organochlorine pesticide release has been banned. Meetings have been arranged with local pest control contractors in an effort to reinforce the new bans and alert them to the problems.

To add to the contamination of fish, *Sydney Morning Herald* 19 October 1989 reports that of the samples of bran tested in 1987 for organophosphate pesticides, 17 out of 17 tested positive to traces of chlorpyrifos-methyl, 21 out of 21 tested positive for fenitrothion and nine tested positive to traces of pirimiphos-methyl.

These organophosphate pesticides, which are extremely toxic nerve poisons, are supposed to break down quickly in the environment, but not fast enough apparently. A number of bran samples also contained traces of the less toxic pyrethroid pesticides and the poisonous heavy metals, lead and cadmium. Analysis of wholemeal bread samples were similar.

'Of the seven samples of peaches tested three contained the persistent organochlorine pesticide dicloran and nine of the 21 sultana samples contained another organochlorine. Six of 14 samples of peanut butter contained heptachlor.'

These results are contained in the still-in-draft-form Market Basket (Noxious Substances) Survey 1987 which is carried out annually but reported on with 'agonising slowness' by the National Health and Medical Research Council (NH & MRC).

The article goes on to say that although the amounts found were small the survey makes it clear that we are ingesting a cocktail of toxic contaminants, many of which accumulate in the body and have the potential to interact with each other thus making them much more poisonous.

It is gratifying to note in this article that a recent test carried out by the New South Wales Department of Health on organically grown fruit and vegetables from a Russells Health Food Store showed NO traces of pesticides for which the Department routinely tests.

Since writing the above I now have a copy of Market Basket Survey 1987. The residue levels in that report of fenitrothion (organophosphate) in bran are 'mean 6.02, median 6.27, 90th percentile 10.09, maximum 12.9 mg/kg'. There are also elevated levels of this pesticide in wholemeal bread and white bread and lower residues in baby cereal. It was noted in the report that fenitrothion was the exception to the low levels of most other pesticide residues and that the organophosphates chlorpyrifos-methyl, fenitrothion and pirimiphos-methyl have shown increases in their detection rates over the period of 1985, 1986 and 1987 surveys.

Organophosphorus nerve poisons were discovered in the 1930s and developed during World War 2 for use in chemical warfare. After the war they were modified and adapted for use as pesticides.

If these extremely toxic nerve poisons are supposedly less residual than the organochlorines, why do we have this increase in residue levels? Have we discarded the organochlorine pesticides in favour of more toxic pesticides which appear also to be residual? I feel we are creating the greatest time bomb the world has ever known.

If these levels of residual chemicals exist in our food chain now, what will be the situation in the years to come if we do not completely stop their usage?

In the light of overwhelming evidence of contamination, it is time that the Australian Standards Association, the Department of Agriculture, local councils throughout Australia and the National Health and Medical Research Council reviewed their registration of chemicals and/or regulations relating to them. For example, in the case of termites, if buildings were constructed to allow for easy inspection on brick piers (with termite capping), or in the case of a slab where the sides are left exposed, together with consideration of the types of timbers to be used, etc, there would not be the necessity for such ground contamination with pesticide sprays. The termite problem does not seem to have been 'solved' by the application of these hazardous chemicals. Surely a building constructed in a way which prevents or deters termites is preferable to such application of these chemicals?

An alternative method of termite control, currently undergoing accreditation to be registered by the Australian Standards Association, is based on a bed of basalt gravel. Trials using this type of gravel (laid on site before construction) to deter subterranean termites have been conducted in Hawaii with 100 per cent success and they are now included in the building code in Hawaii. Short term similar challenge tests have also been conducted by the CSIRO in Melbourne on an Australian species of subterranean termite. These results also confirm the effectiveness of the barrier and suggest that the barrier will be effective permanently. Tests were done on both basalt and granite aggregates, the latter being readily available in Australia as a by-product of concrete manufacture. It is relatively inexpensive given that all indications point to it being permanently effective.

An 'Integrated Termite Management Plan' (which includes site evaluation, building design and construction, etc) is also currently before the Australian Standards Association for approval. These two proposals would eliminate the need for chemical pesticides altogether.

Another system of termite control being considered by the Australian Standards Association is the 'underground pipe connection'. A series of polythene pipes are installed on a bed of sand under the concrete foundation slab. The basic system is similar in principal to an underground sprinkler system. Pesticides are pumped into the system and under pressure the liquid seeps out. However, the system needs refilling every few years. Apparently the system does not require such noxious chemicals as organochlorines. Even so, chemical contamination is becoming such a worldwide problem, surely a method which does not require the use of chemicals at all is preferable.

In a study which came to hand recently, entitled 'Chlorpyrifos in the Ambient Air of Houses Treated for Termites' (C.G. Wright) the findings were unusual. Sixteen houses in North Carolina, United States, were treated sub-soil for termites and air samples taken over a 104 week period. It was interesting to note that residue levels of chlorpyrifos at the 1 week sampling were significantly lower than subsequent sampling and in particular higher residue levels were found in the 52 week samples. The reason for this is unknown. The samples were taken inside the houses and were higher in houses built on sandy soil than those constructed on clay soil, although the type of house construction did not seem to make any significant difference.

All residue levels were lower than the NAS (National Academy of Sciences) interim guideline level of 10 ug/m3 (micrograms per cubic meter). Although the guideline expired in 1985, no new recommendations have been made because sufficient data have not been generated to reassess the original proposed levels. Another point of interest in the study under discussion was that seven of the 16 houses had detectable chlorpyrifos in air samples taken in the living spaces *before* application, although these were very low. The presence of chlorpyrifos in preapplication air samples might have resulted from its earlier use in the houses.

Chlorpyrifos (organophosphate), although initially very poisonous, is considered a less hazardous and less residual termite treatment than the organochlorines, but is it? Healthwise and environmentally, a non-chemical treatment or an 'integrated termite management plan' is the most desirable. Surely then we should be putting all our efforts into the development of safe non-chemical management of pests instead of opting for the 'quick fix'.

Herbicides are another problem in our environment. Research reveals more and more evidence of their harmful effect on our health and the environment. For example, you may remember how my suspected exposure to Amitrole I believe sent me into relapse.

During one of my periods of relapse and recovery I remember listening to a young mother who telephoned a talk-back radio station very concerned as she had just walked into the bedroom where her new baby lay sleeping — in front of an open window — to find a council workman spraying right outside with what she presumed was herbicide. She lived alongside a park. The man was wearing a mask.

The council immediately telephoned the station to say that she had absolutely nothing to worry about — the spray was harmless. However, the following day a spokesman from the NSW Department of Agriculture referred to the matter and was not quite so outspoken about the spray being harmless; rather he said that herbicides should be used with care! A baby weighing just a few kilos would not have anywhere near the resistance of a healthy young adult and even healthy young adults can be adversely affected. I wonder what the long term effects on the delicate immune system of that young baby will be.

When I inquired from NHMRC (Nation Health & Medical Research Council) whether, as well as cancer, testing as to harmful effects on the immune system, or nervous system etc, were also being undertaken, I was told that pesticides, herbicides and other chemicals were constantly being tested and reviewed but that their harmful effects often did not show up until they had been in the community for many years.

It is about time we all spoke up for our right of choice regarding exposure to toxic chemicals and to our absolute right to *clean unpolluted air*.

A landmark case recently on the far north coast may pave the way to stop the large-scale spraying of weeds by councils.

A report in the *Sun Herald* of 5 March 1989 stated

> A retired Sydney University lecturer in histology and embryology, Dr John Pollak, told the court [that] councils and regulatory authorities needed to be more aware of the effects of 2, 4-D on the human immune system. He said plant and animal experiments had revealed 2, 4-D could cause genetic damage, cellular breakdown and retarded growth. 'There is considerable other evidence to suggest that the use of herbicides in general and 2, 4-D in particular should be minimised as much as possible' he told the court.

Where do all these harmful chemicals end up? In our land, rivers, oceans, water and food, the very source of our sustenance and existence.

The toxicity of many pesticides, herbicides and fungicides

The following information is an extract from a booklet entitled 'Agricultural Health' and is reprinted with permission from the Division of Occupational Health — Workers' Compensation and Rehabilitation Authority (previously the NSW Department of Industrial Relations). It sets out the toxicity of many pesticides, herbicides and fungicides in use in Australia today.

Toxicity of many pesticides, herbicides & fungicides

Common name	Trade name	Toxicity to humans (oral and skin contact) (out of 3)
1 Organic phosphates		
Azinphos-ethyl	Gusathion, Benzathion	● ● ●
Azinphos-methyl	Cothion, Gusathion M	● ● ●
Carbophenothion	Trithion	● ● ●
Chlorfenvinphos	Birlane	● ● ●
Chlorpyrifos	Killmaster, Dursban	● ●
Coumaphos	Asuntol	●
Demeton-S-methyl	Metasystox	● ● ●
Diazinon	Gesapon, Neocid	●
Dialifos	Dialifor	● ● ●
Dichlorvos	Nuvan, Mafu	● ● ●
Dicrotophos	Bidrin	● ● ●
Dimefox	Pestox	● ● ●
Dioxathion	Delnav	● ● ●
Dimethoate	Rogor	● ●
Disulfoton	Disyston	● ● ●
Ethion	Ethion	● ● ●
Ethoprophos	Prophos	● ● ●
Famphur	Warbex	● ● ●
Fenamiphos	Nemacur	● ● ●
Fenthion	Lebaycid	● ●
Fenthion ethyl	Lucijet	● ● ●
Fenitrothion	Sumithion	● ●
Fensulfothion	Dasanit	● ● ●

Common name	Trade name	Toxicity (out of 3)
Hexaethyl tetraphosphate	TEPP	•••
Isocarbophos, isofenphos	BAY SRA	•••
Leptophos	Phosvel	•••
Maldison	Malathion	•
Mecarbam	Murfotox	•••
Methamidophos	Tamaron	•••
Methidathion	Supracide	•••
Mevinphos	Phosdrin	•••
Mipafox	Pestox	••
Monocrotophos	Azodrin, Nuvacron	•••
Napthalophos	Rametin-H	•••
Omethoate	Folimat	•••
Parathion	Folidol E605	•••
Parathion-methyl	Folidol M50	•••
Phenkapton	—	•••
Phorate	Thimet	•••
Phosphamidon	Dimecron	•••
Schradan	Dimefox	•••
Sulfotep	Bladafum	•••
Terbufos		•••
Trichlorphon	Dipterex	•

2 Carbamates

Common name	Trade name	Toxicity (out of 3)
Aldicarb	Temik	•••
Aminocarb	Metacil	•••
Bendiocarb	Ficam	•••
Carbaryl	7Sevin	•••
Carbofuran	Furadan	•••
Formetanate		•••
Methomyl	Lannate	•••
Oxamyl	Vydate	•••
Promecarb	Carbamult	•••

Common name	Trade name	Toxicity (out of 3)
Propoxur	Baygon	● ● ●
Thiofanox	Decamox	● ● ●

3 *Chlorinated hydrocarbons (organochlorines)*

Common name	Trade name	Toxicity
Aldrin	Aldrex	● ● ●
Camphechlor	Toxaphene	● ●
Chlordane	Chlordane	● ●
D.D.T.	D.D.T.	● ●
Dieldrin	Dieldrex	● ● ●
Endosulfan	Thiodan	● ● ●
Endrin	Endrin	● ● ●
Heptachlor	Heptachlor HC 80	● ● ●
Lindane	Commexane	● ● ●

4 *Herbicides and fungicides*

Common name	Trade name	Toxicity
Acrolein	Aqualin	● ● ●
Aminotriazole	Amitrole, Weedazole Cammellia	●
Arsenic (inorganic)	Sodium arsenate	● ● ●
Atrazine	Gesaprim	●
Bromacil	Hyvar	●
Captan	Captan	●
Bromoxynil	Brominil Weedoban	●
Di-Nitro, orthocresol	DNCO	● ● ●
Dioseb	D.N.B.P.	● ● ●
2,4-D	2,4-D	●
Diquat	Reglone	● ● ●
Paraquat	Gramoxone	● ● ●
Pentachlorphenol	Pentabrite, Santabride	● ●
2,4,5-T	2,4,5-T	●

Common name	Trade name	Toxicity (out of 3)
5 Others		
Arsenic trioxide	—	●●●
Chlordimeform	CGS 500	●●●
Cyhalothrin	New Product	●●
Deltamethrin	Clout, Decamethrin	●●

●●● Extremely Toxic   ●● Toxic   ● Moderate or Low Toxicity

Suspect Carcinogenic Materials

The following are classified as industrial substances suspected of carcinogenic potential for humans:

Arsenic pentoxide	Dieldrin
Arsenic trioxice	DSMA
Carbon tetrachloride	Ethylene dibromide
Camphechlor	Ethylene oxide
Captan	Heptachlor
CDEC	Lead arsenate
Chlordane	Lindane
Chlordimeform	MSMA
Copper chrome arsenate	Sodium arsenate
(CCA timber treatment)	Sulfallate
DDT	

Arsenic and chromium compounds have carcinogenic potential.

Although the acute toxicity of some of these compounds is low, exposure should be avoided or reduced to a low level because of suspected carcinogenic properties.

Ethylene dibromide used as an agricultural and horticultural fumigant for soil and plants must be used with extreme care.

My thanks to the Division of Occupational Health for their assistance.

If exposure to pesticide and herbicide sprays is a problem to you as it is to me, may I suggest that the following approach worked for me.

First, get a certificate from your doctor, or clinical ecologist, to the effect that you have a severe sensitivity to pesticides, herbicides, etc and that exposure to these chemicals will cause relapse. Write a letter to your local council enclosing the certificate requesting that they notify you if they intend spraying in the area so that you can vacate if necessary. If this brings no result, legal action can be taken, provided you have medical back-up and your claims are genuine. Claims for compensation may bring about changes.

Second, notify all your neighbours about your problem. Request them to notify you if they are having any treatment undertaken on their property which may result in a 'drift' over your property or which is close enough to your property for you to inhale the fumes. Some pesticides have a very strong odour (eg chlordane, heptachlor) which stay around for a long time. Again claims for compensation may bring about changes provided they are genuine.

In the main I have found people very willing to help me avoid sprays provided I took the opportunity to alert them to the dangers.

I will do anything to stay well!

Other toxic chemicals

Besides pesticides and herbicides we are hit by a barrage of other toxic chemicals. These fall into several other categories including petrochemicals, formaldehyde, volatile aromatic solvents and volatile chlorinated solvents.

Phenol-Carbolic acid

Phenol is obtained from benzene and toluene by various chemical processes. Phenol is known to be toxic to the nervous system and some research has also implicated phenols as cofactors in the origin of certain types of cancers.

Exposure to phenol sends me into relapse very quickly and causes my body to burn with hot-ice type pins and needles just under the skin. It has, in my observations, been involved in my relapses to a large extent, but not all of them. I would really like to see more research done into the effects of this widely used product on the human body and the immune sytem. It is poisonous and may cause death if swallowed.

It is used in the manufacture of phenolic and epoxy resins for plastics, weed killers, germicidal paints, pharmaceuticals, preservatives, aspirin, allergy antigen serum, nylon, pesticides, polyurethane, photography solutions, bakelite moulded articles, synthetic detergents, perfumes, petrol, dyes, antiseptics and disinfectants, processed foods and is contained in cigarette smoke — to name but a few sources. Cans of tinned foods, except edible oils, are lined with an epoxyphenolic lining.

Formaldehyde

Formaldehyde, a colourless gas with a stifling odour, is found in so many products. It was discovered in 1867 by August Wilhelm von Hofmann, a German Scientist, and was mainly used to preserve insects and other biological specimens. However, it is now used in a seemingly endless number of products including embalming preparations, antiseptics, disinfectants, antibiotics, germicidal soaps, cosmetics, antiperspirants, shampoos, mouthwashes, insecticides, rat poisons, concrete, plaster, wallboard, synthetic resins and dyes. Urea-formaldehye and phenol-formaldehyde resins are used as glues and laminating agents in plywood and particle board, foam plastic, and urea foam insulation in walls and ceilings. It is also used to make fabrics shrink-proof, crease-resistant, dye-fast, flame-resistant and mothproof. Formaldehyde is used as a finish for carpets, and to improve the strength and water resistance of paper products.

As you can see, it is used in just about everything we come in contact with in everyday living: our houses, our workplace, our cosmetics, our clothes and in some medications and vitamin preparations. It is rather difficult to avoid. In moderate concentrations it causes watery, sore eyes, and nose irritation and inflammation. In high concentrations it can cause inflamed eyes, sore throats, bronchitis, asthma and skin rashes. The effects of long-term exposure to low levels are unknown, however it has caused cancer of the nose in rats and a leading Sydney clinical ecologist tells me that it suppresses the immune system. It causes me to get a sore nose and throat immediately at moderate to high concentrations, and prolonged exposure sends me into relapse. It is second on the list after natural gas as a common cause of allergies. (Dr Mackarness — *Chemical Victims*).

Volatile Aromatic Solvents and Volatile Chlorinated Solvents

(Benzene, Toluene, Ethylbenzene, Xylenes, Styrene, and Trimethylbenzenes).

(Dichloromethane, Chloroform, 1,1,1 Trichloroethane, Trichloroethylene, Perchlorethylene, Tetrachloroethylene, Dichlorbenzenes.)

These solvents are used in hundreds of industrial processes and thousands of consumer products including paints, stains, glues, napthalene (moth balls), polishes, cleaners, detergents, pesticides, perfumes, disinfectant, polyesters, paint strippers, pharmaceuticals, dry cleaning agents, deodorants, moth proofing, water proofing, silicon sprays and floor polishes. Mineral turpentine is a derivative of benzene.

THERE ARE NO KNOWN OR PROVEN SAFE LEVELS OF THESE SOLVENTS.

They can cause central nervous system depression (headaches, fatigue, nausea, respiratory failure, behaviour disorders or impaired co-ordination); mucosa and skin irritations (conjunctivitis, corneal erosion, dermatitis, asthma, bronchitis); they are toxic to the liver and kidneys and there is a possibility of chromosomal defects. Glue sniffing can cause permanent brain damage. Benzene is a known and proven cause of cancer. Products containing these solvents are freely available at the stores and there does not appear to be enough warning of the real dangers of ingestion, inhalation or skin absorption. Certainly the general public has not been made aware of the hazards associated with these solvents. According to a highly qualified lecturer in nursing and midwifery, and the Sydney Poisons Information Service, napthalene (a derivative of benzene) can cause headaches, nausea and vomiting. One moth ball swallowed by a small child can make it extremely ill and precipitate convulsions. Napthalene can also cause blood disorders in babies and children who lack an enzyme called glucose six phosphate dehydrogenase; however, it is not emphasised that napthalene should not be used near them.

I was told recently of a child who developed aplastic anaemia. She lived alongside a service station. The specialist treating her seemed to think there was a connection between the benzene and other toxic chemicals emanating from the service station and her disease. He advised them to move.

PCBs or Plasticisers

PCBs are now banned. They include a group of 209 possible isomers of unsubstituted biphenyls. PCBs were developed as a coolant for electrical transformers. They were previously found in heat transfer fluids, hydraulic fluids, lubricants, plasticisers, coatings, inks, carbonless copy paper, pesticides and other products.

They have a low order of acute toxicity but because of their high fat solubility, poor metabolism and indefinite half-life the problems with bio-accumulation are great. A major target organ of PCB contamination is the liver. PCBs are potent enzyme inducers and they decrease thiamine levels in blood and liver and elevate triglycerides.

Pentachlorophenol

Is used as a wood preservative, in anti-microbal preparations and defoliants. It is acquired by ingestion, inhalation and dermal absorption of powders and solutions.

Blood Tests

It was not until I had almost finished writing this book that I discovered blood testing for selected chemicals was available in USA. (Doctors who arrange these tests are listed in the Directory page 206.)

Organochlorine pesticides, aromatic and chlorinated solvents, PCBs and pentachlorophenol accumulate in the fatty tissue and according to Dr Eric can be picked up in blood tests as they are continually leaking into the bloodstream. When (due to illness or some other cause, such as fasting) weight loss occurs, they can be released into the bloodstream in quite significant quantities. At the time my blood was taken (June 1989) I was in a very good state of health and was not under weight.

The results, I believe, more than prove that I have very high levels of organochlorine pesticides and pentachlorophenol as well as some aromatic and chlorinated solvents. This would, in my opinion, seem to bear out my contention that they are a major cause of my illness.

Summary of my tests

Organochlorine pesticides

Primary problems would appear to be organochlorines with HCBs (hexachlorobenzene) approximately 100 times the US average. The DDE/DDT group is approximately 8–10 times higher, and the DIELDRIN level slightly raised. (I have no known exposure to HCB which was discontinued in the early '80s. It was used extensively as a fungicide in the wheat industry and has high residual properties. Nor have I any known exposure to DDE/DDT).

Volatile aromatic hydrocarbons
Toluene, Xylenes and Styrene are significantly raised.

Volatile chlorinated hydrocarbons
The levels of chloroform, 1,1,1, Trichlorethane, Tetrachloroethylene and Dichloromethane are all significantly raised.

Pentachlorophenol
Pentachlorophenol, a general biocide, is twice the US average.

In summary, overall markedly high levels of a large number of compounds in the blood demonstrate failure of body clearance and/or high exposure to chemicals.

On the next page is a graph of my blood test results, compared to the US population (normalised figures).

Dr Mark Donohue and Dr Joachim Fluhrer, have referred over 300 ME/CFS sufferers to have the tests for toxic chemicals in their blood. Their results are remarkably similar to mine and, what is even more alarming, they too have found *much higher* levels than in the United States — up to ten times as great.

The following charts, drawn from figures provided by Dr Donohue, show the ME/CFS average for Australia and the normal average for the US, and show clear comparisons between the two countries. The results for Australia were averages from 96 blood specimens of ME/CFS patients as at January 1989.

Toxic chemical levels in author's blood samples compared to US population

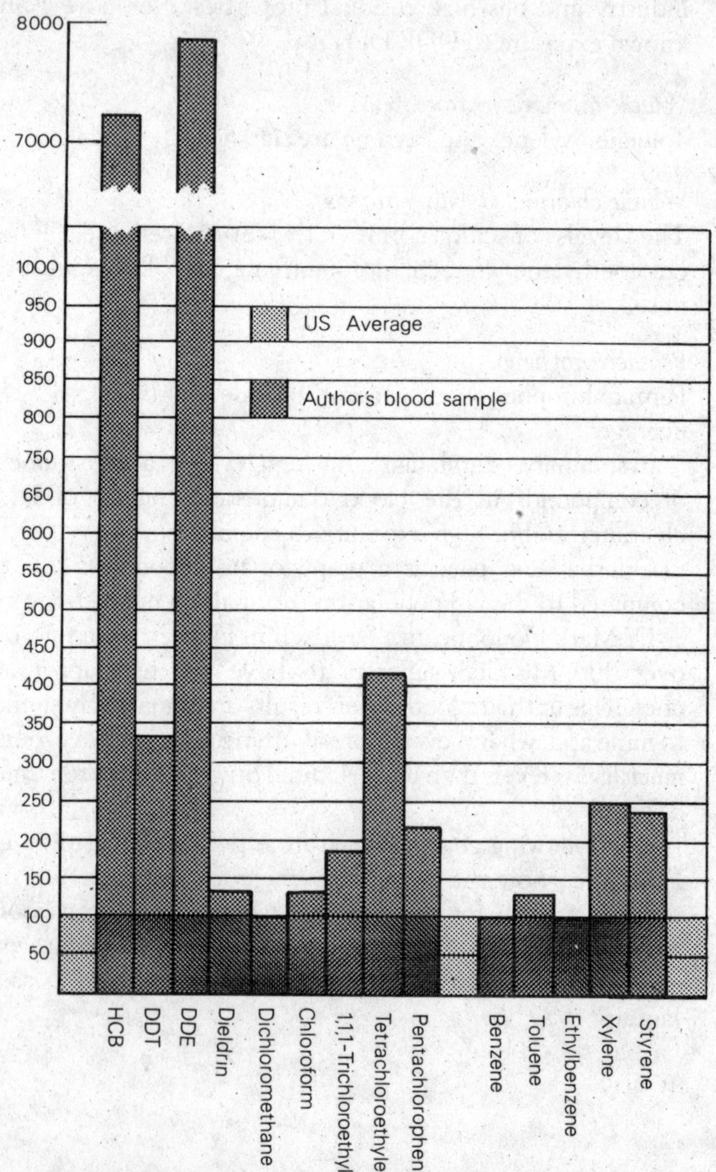

Toxic chemical levels in Australian ME/CFS blood samples compared to US population

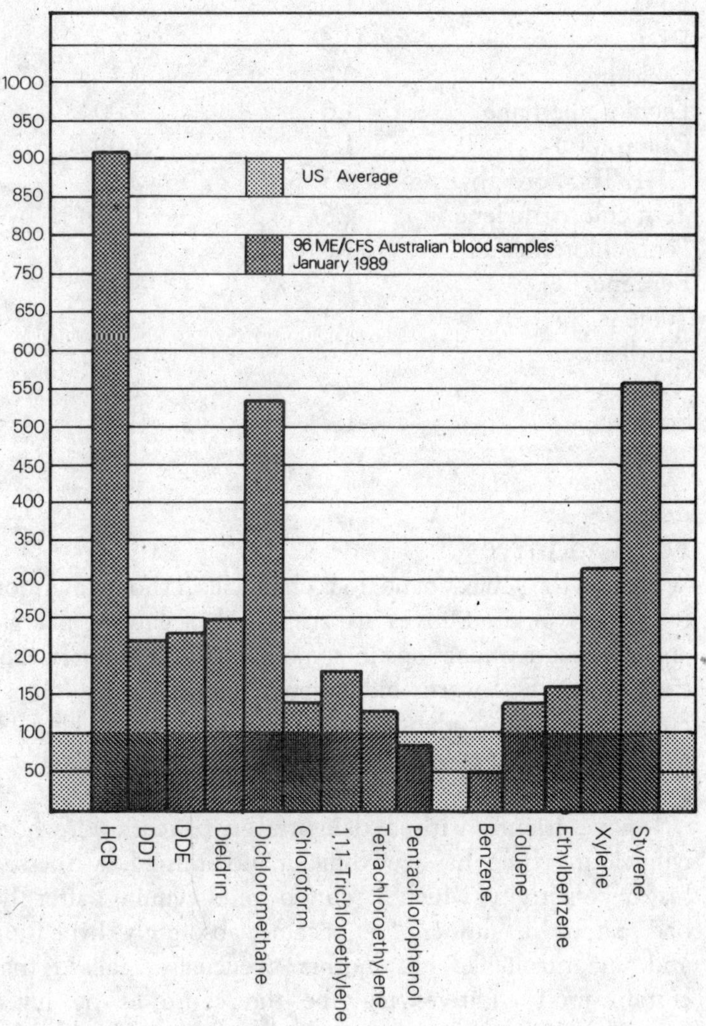

My *actual* results, in parts per billion, compared to the US average, are given below.

	My results	US Average
HCB	21.2	0.3
DDT	1.0	0.3
DDE	44.5	5.6
Dieldrin	0.4	0.3
Dichloromethane	1.0	1.00
Chloroform	1.3	1.00
1,1,1, Trichloroethylene	0.5	0.5
Tetrachloroethylene	4.6	1.1
Pentachlorophenol	11.0	5.0
Benzene	1.0	1.0
Toluene	1.2	0.9
Ethylbenzene	0.5	1.0
Xylenes	2.5	1.0
Styrene	1.2	0.5

Food additives

Whilst on the subject of noxious chemicals, I should mention that many food additives are suspected of causing allergic and hyperactive reactions in some adults and children. For example Dr Eric warns his patients against buying 'chips'. Apparently anti-oxidants are often added to cooking oil which is being re-used and these can trigger off asthma and other allergies.

I have friends with a delightful two year old whose behaviour at times has been difficult and unusual. I witnessed his hyperactivity which occurred one evening after he had eaten his dinner. He became absolutely hyped up and uncontrollable. His mother eventually realised that certain food additives may be the cause as he loved commercially-produced sauces and sausages. He was not given any commercially-produced products for a week or so and the change in his behaviour was really remarkable.

What behavioural patterns indicate *hyperactivity* as against *normal* activity in children and adults? The Hyperactivity Association of Chatswood, New South Wales, describes them as follows.

Marked hyperactivity — rocks, jiggles legs, dances, wiggles hands (this *may* be manifested by crib rocking and head banging in infancy) tears around like a lunatic, cannot keep still.

Compulsive aggression — disruptive at school, will not conform to normal discipline, touches everything and everyone, cannot be diverted from actions.

Excitable, impulsive — behaviour is unpredictable, panics easily with temper tantrums, demands must be met immediately, cries often and easily.

Short attention span — flits from one project to another, unable to concentrate or sit through lessons, meals, TV programme, etc.

Exceptionally clumsy.

Poor muscle co-ordination. Eyes and hands do not seem to function together, difficulty with buttons, writing, drawing and playground activity.

Poor sleeping habits, woken easily.

Normal IQ.

It is interesting that boys are much more affected than girls.

This syndrome is not confined to children but can affect adults in the same way. Nor is it triggered by food additives only. It can be triggered by strong chemical smells including paints, perfumes, sprays etc. In other words it would appear to be an allergic reaction of the brain to substances the body just cannot tolerate. Consider the adult with this hypersensitivity syndrome, possessed by driven behaviour and very little self-control.

There are many experts who maintain that our diet and physical environment govern our health and behaviour. I would have to agree.

My thanks to the Hyperactivity Association of NSW for supplying the information regarding symptoms of hyperactivity and the following food additives to be avoided together with their codes.

Colourings

102	Tartrasine — yellow colour
107	Yellow 2G
110	Sunset Yellow FCF
122	Carmoisine — red colour
123	Amaranth — red colour
124	Ponceau 4 R — red colour
127	Erythrosine — cherry pink to red colour
132	Indigotine — blue colour
133	Brilliant blue
142	Green S
151	Brilliant Black
155	Brown HT
160b	Annatto — yellow to peach or red colour

Preservatives

200	Sorbic acid	
201	Sodium sorbate	Sorbic Acids
202	Potassium sorbate	
203	Calcium sorbate	
210	Benzoic acid	
211	Sodium benzoate	Benzoic Acids
212	Potassium benzoate	
213	Calcium benzoate	
220	Sulphur dioxide	
221	Sodium sulphite	
222	Sodium bisulphite	Sulphites
223	Sodium metabisulphite	
224	Potassium metabisulphite	

249   Potassium nitrite } Nitrites
250   Sodium nitrite   }
251   Sodium nitrate   } Nitrates
252   Potassium nitrate }

Anti-oxidants
310   Propyl gallate
311   Octyl gallate
312   Dodecyl gallate
320   Butylated hydroxyanisole (BHA)
321   Butylated hydroxytoluene (BHT)

Glutamates
620   L-Glutamic acid
621   Monosodium glutamate (MSG)
622   Monopotassium glutamate
623   Calcium dihydrogen di-L-glutamate

The dietitian at the Royal Prince Alfred Hospital, Sydney, adds further possible problem areas:

319   tert-Butylhydroquinone (TBHQ) — antioxidant
216   Propyl 4-hydroxybenzoate
218   Methyl 4-hydroxybenzoate

(Both 216 and 218 are only permitted for use with artifical colours which are already listed above).

627   Disodium guanylate
631   Disodium inosinate

(Both 627 and 631 have not been added to the Australian list but are presently under investigation).

As these food additives have the potential to trigger off allergic reactions in chemically sensitive people it would be wise for ME/CFS sufferers to avoid them. We seem to have progressed a long way down the track since the days of preserving with sugar, salt and vinegar.

For further information on this subject I would recommend

The New Additive Code Breaker by Maurice Hanssen with Jill Marsden, revised for Australia by Betty Norris. The possible harmful effects of many other food additives are covered in this book.

Heavy metals

An acquaintance who has been very sick with ME/CFS for a few years telephoned me the other day, so excited, as she has improved radically since having her amalgam fillings systematically removed by the dentist recently. She has lost most of the bizarre symptoms of head pain she had been experiencing and is sure she is on the road to recovery. She is convinced she has been suffering from mercury poisoning!

I mention this because, added to the noxious chemicals bombarding us, is a build up of mercury, lead, cadmium and (although not a heavy metal) aluminium. That is not to say that everyone should rush out and have their fillings replaced with an inert material as I know of sufferers who have done just that, but alas it has not effected a cure. Perhaps in my acquaintance's case the mercury levels were higher than normal and added to all the other toxins she had absorbed, that was the catalyst to her total relapse. She is also of the opinion that the metal fillings affected the electrical charges in her body and contributed to dizziness and pain.

Mercury is found in our fish and shellfish particularly. As it is used in the manufacture of various products including paint, organomercurial fungicides, pulp, cosmetics and electrical products, it is entering our environment as a waste product thus leading to the contamination of our water and food supply. Mercury loss occurs from amalgam fillings over a period of time adding yet another poisonous substance our body has to cope with.

Years ago we were alerted to the dangers of lead paint. But lead is still building up in our environment, mostly as a result of petrol driven vehicles. Although lead-free petrol is now available, it will be a long time before all the vehicles using leaded petrol are off the roads. Lead fallout accumulates in the environment. It does not break down, but is absorbed by crops, livestock and by us. Children are particularly vulnerable from vehicle exhaust fumes and higher levels of lead have been found in crops growing close to the road. Thus we are creating the build up of another poisonous metal in our environment.

Now, add to all that, aluminium. Aluminium was thought to be harmless and has been put to an endless number of uses including food packaging and cooking utensils. Aluminium cannot be mined as a pure metal but is mined as bauxite. It is recovered from bauxite by an electrochemical treatment which uses vast amounts of electric power. There is evidence linking high levels of aluminium in brain tissue with Alzheimer's Disease. Some antacid preparations contain aluminium and Dr Eric does not recommend them, also some infant milk formulas and intravenous fluids have been found to contain high levels of aluminium.

In conclusion then I can only say *be careful*! As is obvious from the foregoing the real problems in our mass-production, greedy society are only now really becoming apparent. I am sure that, of the many chemicals used over the years, the manufacturers were as innocent regarding their hazardous health effects as were the consumers. However, this cannot be said in all cases. Not enough testing has been done and much information has been withheld from the general public. We are all too trusting.

Therefore, be diligent, ask now that manufacturers guarantee the safety of their products and insist on adequate labelling. The consumer can begin to rectify some of these problems by trying not to purchase doubtful or toxic products. The manufacturers will soon get the message.

5   The problem with water

Unfortunately man has not considered the long-term effects of his abuse of our world and we cannot now be fully guaranteed that our drinking water is uncontaminated. Pesticides, herbicides and other toxic wastes used in suburban and agricultural spraying end up in our waterways. Add to that the artificial fertilisers which are upsetting the balance of nature and the toxic fumes in the air which are continually falling to earth, and you can see it is a problem of huge dimensions and needs a very quick solution.

There are about 50 chemicals which have been approved by the National Health and Medical Research Council for use in our water supply but only a few are regularly used. The most common include chlorine, fluoride, ammonia and occasionally aluminium sulphate. Ammonia was added three to four years ago in Sydney, to combine with chlorine and form chloramine thus making the chlorine, which rids the water of algae, bacteria and moulds, more effective to carry 'all the way to the tap' and to stop the formation of by-products such as trihalomethanes and organochlorines. Obviously if the water supply was not disinfected we would all be extremely ill due to infection, however, in the disinfection process we seem to be creating another set of problems. As we are all of differing metabolisms there are people who are allergic to the various chemical additives, and notice an improvement in their health once they drink only purified water. Chlorinated drinking water is now being linked to coronary disease.

The question of fluoridation has been debated at length but data which has come to light in recent years would indicate that it may do more harm than good. The fundamental fact which has been overlooked is that we are being compulsorily 'dosed' with something which will not benefit the whole of the population (particularly older people and those with false teeth) and which has been linked to RSI (repetitive strain injury), mottled teeth (dental flurosis) and now cancer. Chlorine is used to treat the *water* (and the by-products of this have caused other problems), however, fluoride is added to treat *people*. There is a fundamental difference between the two and we should have a 'choice' in the matter.

For those who feel they 'need' fluoride, toothpaste and tablets are readily available. This way the dose can be controlled as it is virtually impossible to ensure that each person receives the individual correct 'dose' from the tap especially when they are ingesting fluoride from other sources as well. Fluoride is contained in most foods and is particularly high in tea, seafood, bone meal, spinach and gelatin. Some plants such as spinach, lettuce and parsley are fluoride accumulators.

And there is some doubt about its efficacy. A recent survey of two major capital cities of Australia revealed that children drinking unfluoridated water had better teeth than those drinking fluoridated water! Austria, Belgium, Denmark, France, Greece, Holland, Italy, Luxembourg, Norway, Spain, Sweden, West Germany and Yugoslavia have rejected fluoridation and so have hundreds of cities in the USA. Less than eight per cent of Britain's population drinks fluoridated water.

Of course the argument is that fluoride occurs *naturally* in some water. The fact that fluoride occurs in water which contains a high content of calcium and magnesium (ie *hard water*) has been overlooked. Calcium negates the toxic effects of fluoride. Therefore we are again tampering with nature and this invariably ends in disaster.

In his book *Food Chemical Sensitivity* Dr Robert Buist (PhD) quotes the conclusions of a report submitted by Philip Sutton, Academic Associate at the University of Melbourne, in 1980, to the Committee of Inquiry into the Fluoridation of Victorian Water Supplies. Of the twenty-four summarised conclusions there is very little evidence to support artificial fluoridation. In fact he concludes that ten per cent of children who drink fluoridated water from birth will develop dental fluorosis due to fluoride poisoning of toothforming cells. There are people who are sensitive to it and whose health improves once they lower their consumption of fluoride. Preliminary data from Birmingham, England strongly supports a link to cancer. Also, there is little known about the effects on the central nervous system, or the brain and, as it may affect the kidneys, should not be used in dialysis machines.

When so many countries have rejected it, why are we compulsorily dosing our population? Even though I have a water purifier, I cannot avoid watering my vegetables with fluoride! We should have a choice. My husband was medically diagnosed as having been overdosed with fluoride. This occurred after a visit to the dentist when fluoride was applied to his teeth. He used fluoride toothpaste and was drinking fluoridated water.

Tank water

If you have a tank, make sure it can be hooked up to the collection area only after it has been raining for some considerable time, so that all the pollution which has fallen onto the collection area can be washed away before the water is collected in the tank. This will not eliminate all the pollutants, as many toxic chemicals are contained in the rain itself from chimneys belching forth exhaust fumes, aerial spraying and crop dusting, etc. Traces of radiation fallout were found in Canada a few days after the Chernobyl disaster which will give you an indication of just how far aerial toxic waste travels.

It is interesting to note that when I tested both a tank on the mid-north coast and a tank on the outskirts of Sydney, the PH level was 7.0 and 6.8 respectively. (The higher the PH level the less the acidity.) 5.6 is considered 'acid rain' and is falling in parts of Europe well below that level. Australia is in a unique position as we do not have so much heavy industry on our doorstep. That should not make us complacent however.

It is wise to boil tank water before drinking and to be aware of the cleanliness and composition of the collection area. Roofs painted with toxic paints (e.g. old lead-based paints), asbestos roofs, PVC pipes etc, should not be used for water collection. The manufacturers of various roofing products will advise as to the toxicity of the materials and in this regard I found Lysaght Building Industries, Sydney, very helpful. The CSIRO have information on many products and problems.

Water Purifiers

There are three types of water filters which work as follows:

1 activated carbon
2 ion exchange resins
3 reverse osmosis

Water distillation is the other method of purification, however it is a lengthy process.

About two years ago I purchased an 'All Pure' water purifier from a health food store. It had two types of cartridges contained in the cylinder: one contained ion exchange resins and the other activated carbon. I experienced quite a deal of trouble with it as the water would 'go off' and smell like dead fish after a very short space of time. As the cartridges were expensive and I seemed to be making regular trips to the store, the distributors stood by their product, changed the resins free of charge until I was satisfied and eventually changed the purifier completely. In the meantime the manufacturer discarded the activated carbon filter and now relies solely on ion exchange resins. I have had no further trouble. However, I have since spoken to a water expert at the Sydney Water Board who told me that often the carbon attracts moulds and bacteria and this could have accounted for the problem.

According to the May 1989 edition of CHOICE magazine, the 'All Pure' purifier tested well, is reasonably priced and the cartridges are slightly cheaper than the comparable type purifier 'Testa' which performed somewhat better. This type of purifier removes most types of harmful chemicals including pesticides, chlorine and fluoride but does not remove bacteria which can easily be removed by boiling.

There was not a significant difference in the chemical performance of the reverse osmosis systems except that some removed the bacteria, but as they are slow to operate, and waste water, I personally cannot see the advantage. CHOICE gives a very good comparison of water purifiers.

According to CHOICE there was no easy way of testing to see if the filters were still working efficiently however, I was supplied with a bottle of testing fluid at the time of purchase, and was told that the water would acquire a slight 'bad fish' smell when the resins needed replacing. This is indeed what happened.

Another survey was conducted by the magazine *Simply Living*. This passed as 100 per cent effective all those purifiers with reverse osmosis and covered a wider range of chemicals than did CHOICE. However they made no comparison of the time it took to filter the water which was certainly much longer with the reverse osmosis process — up to 20 minutes per glass in some purifiers. The 'Testa' performed as for *CHOICE* although it did not eliminate the additional chemicals tested by *Simply Living* such as nitrate, sulphate, free residual chloride, PCBs and DDT.

The best of the ion exchange type resin filters was 'Creative Purifiers' but it is comparatively more expensive. This purifier was not included in the *CHOICE* survey.

I would certainly recommend obtaining a copy of *CHOICE* May 1989 and *Simply Living* Vol. 3, Number 9, if you wish to investigate further.

Another purifier which was not included in either of the above surveys is Cartier. This company claims their mid-range purifier performs as well as the 'Creative Purifier' which is similarly priced. Cartier have a larger range of water purifiers. If you wish to follow this up you'll find Cartier's address in the directory (page 224).

In order to save space, I attach my purifier to the bath tap and stand the purifier in the bath. It is close to the kitchen and does not take up space on the kitchen bench. If the laundry is more convenient, use that. Remember to use only cold water through the purifier.

If the quality of your water supply is of concern to you we found that the Water Board will test it for chlorine and other chemical residues. Perhaps it was just coincidence, but the quality of our water improved dramatically afterwards.

6   The harm of cigarette smoke

Before I realised what was contributing to my illness I spent the evening in a room with half a dozen smokers. The smell of cigarette smoke has bothered me for a good number of years, long before I became ill, but, in order to comply with the social graces I did not complain. As I had been exposed to pesticide the week previously and was gradually deteriorating, this particular evening was the final straw to a complete relapse. It was at this stage, in 1985, that Dr Eric realised my problem revolved around toxic chemicals. This was the key factor in determining my future course of action and thus making some real headway in regaining my health, and staying well.

Smoking falls into two categories: *mainstream* (direct inhalation of smoke by smokers) and *sidestream* (indirect inhalation of smoke by non-smokers). Passive, or sidestream, smoking is also called 'involuntary smoking' because non-smokers do not usually choose to breathe smoke polluted air. As a matter of principle, I belive that smoking control policies should try to ensure that smokers maintain their freedom to smoke provided this does not infringe on the rights of non-smokers to breathe smoke-free air, though one might also argue that no-one has the right to pollute the air wittingly.

Here is a breakdown of selected toxic and carcinogenic

smoke constituents in sidestream and mainstream smoke as supplied by the 'Quit for Life' programme NSW Department of Health.

Please note that as variable figures were supplied for ammonia and hydrogen cyanide, in order to simplify the matter I have taken an average.

Ratio of Concentration

Constituents	Sidestream/Mainstream
1 Carbon monoxide	8:1
2 Ammonia	8:1
3 Hydrogen cyanide	0.25:1
4 Formaldehyde (inhibits lungcilia)	51:1
5 Acrolein	12:1
6 3-Vinylpyridine	28:1
7 Nicotine	3:1
8 Toluene	5.6:1
9 Phenol	2.6:1
10 Napthalene	16:1
11 Benzo (a) pyrene (Carcinogen)	3:1
12 B-Napthylamine (Carcinogen)	39:1
13 Dimethyl Nitrosamine (Carcinogen)	52:1
14 4-Amino Byphenyl (Carcinogen)	30:1

As you can see from the above sidestream smoke contains more of these chemicals than mainstream smoke.

Note also that three quarters of the nicotine contained in a filter cigarette is liberated into the air by way of sidestream smoke. Nicotine is more acutely toxic, on a weight for weight basis, than either arsenic or cyanide.

Add to those components pesticide (as most crops are sprayed liberally) which is released by way of smoke, and thus inhaled.

Cigarette smoking also produces carbon monoxide, which can be very dangerous. We have just recently seen the untimely death of young children travelling from the country in a van which allowed carbon monoxide fumes to penetrate. The family became sleepy, and because carbon monoxide is colourless, odourless and tasteless, no-one realised the danger. Some of them have sadly perished.

Carbon monoxide is strongly attracted to the red blood cells (haemoglobin) and renders them unable to carry oxygen to the muscles. As the red blood cells take up to 140 days to be excreted from the body (they are being replaced all the time) they 'rattle around' in the blood stream 'paralysed' and unable to carry vital oxygen to the muscles, resulting, of course, in lethargy and tiredness.

These facts were supplied to me by Dr Rene Bittoun who runs the very successful St Vincents Hospital Smokers Clinic in Sydney.

It is no wonder, then, that ME/CFS sufferers are affected by cigarette smoke. As mentioned in the first chapter, Dr Mukherjee's studies of ME/CFS sufferers found that in relapse the red blood cells change shape and stiffen thus making it difficult for them to quickly travel through the small capillaries and veins, thereby affecting the supply of oxygen to the muscles. Combined with the effects of cigarette smoke one could expect to get a 'double barrel' problem. Maybe this is an explanation for our resulting fatigue or relapse.

(I have noticed that ME/CFS sufferers who smoke do not seem to be as aware of, or sensitive to, toxic chemicals. Perhaps they *are* sensitive and the constant ingestion of chemicals by way of cigarette smoke is masking their problems, which, unrecognised, is aggravating and prolonging their illness, in much the same way as eating food regularly to which one has become allergic will mask that allergy.)

Apart from formaldehyde and phenol, which were discussed in the chapter on pesticides and herbicides, cigarette smoke also contains toluene, a solvent similar to benzene. There are no known safe levels of these solvents.

They are toxic to the liver and can cause a significant number of symptoms similar to ME/CFS. I have listed a few of the toxic chemicals contained in cigarette smoke to give you an idea of why, like myself, everyone is very adversely affected by it. Needless to say, one can understand how smoking causes cancer and why it is a very undesirable habit to pursue. It is most gratifying to find that at last there are places one can visit without being subjected to cigarette smoke and that the government and employers are making a real effort to clean up the workplace.

Maybe the chemical additives in present-day cigarettes are more of a problem than the old-fashioned roll-your-own cigarettes made from organically-grown tobacco!

*   *   *

Since writing this chapter and the publication of the first edition of my book, toxicology reports have come to hand which contain the most alarming information as to the effects on blood, bone marrow and the immune system generally, of certain drugs, pesticides, herbicides, benzene, toluene, phenol, glycol ethers and many other toxic chemicals in general use. The United States Department of Health has been researching such effects over a period of years and their findings between 1983–86 are summed up as follows:

> Chemicals of environmental concern have been shown to induce immunosuppression as evidenced by altered antibody-mediated immunity, cell-mediated immunity, natural killer cell activity or macrophage function in rodents following sublethal exposure. Some examples of chemical immunotoxicants include asbestos, polyhalogenated aromatic hydrocarbons, diethylstilbenstrol, polycyclic aromatic hydrocarbons, hexachlorobenzene, pentachlorophenol and certain organo and heavy metals. Studies have also indicated that exposure to certain chemicals can alter host resistance to bacteria, viruses,

parasites and transplanted tumor cells ... Three classes of undesirable effects may occur when the immune system is perturbed by advertent (eg, drugs) or inadvertent (eg, environmental pollutants) exposure to chemicals and include: (1) those which result in immunodeficiency or suppresion; (2) those which alter host defence mechanisms; and (3) those which induce hypersensitivity or allergy.

(Dr M. Luster, PhD, *National Toxicology Program*, US Department of Health and Human Services, p. 171)

Also the research findings contained in 'Environmentally Related Disorders of the Hematologic and Immune Systems' by Michael I. Luster, PhD, Daniel Wierda, PhD and Gary J. Rosenthal PhD (*Medical Clinics of North America* Vol 74, No. 2 March 1990) show further evidence of the effects of drugs and environmental chemicals on bone marrow and blood cell counts (eg benzene and aplastic anaemia) not to mention the various pesticides and drugs cited therein adversely affecting the nervous system and immune system. Yet we are expected to believe that small amounts of pesticides are harmless (even though they quickly kill insects and small living creatures and are residual) that drugs are the only answer to our illnesses (when in fact they often depress the immune system) and that homoeopathy and herbal remedies are either ineffective or poisonous. Where is the logic in these arguments?

III   *Cure and prevention*

7   Homoeopathy, naturopathy and herbalism

Homoeopathy

Homoeopathic treatment uses over 6000 substances, called 'remedies', culled from a wide range of plant, animal, mineral and other sources. These substances are prepared through a careful series of dilutions and shaking. The three basic principles of homoeopathy state that:

1 it is the constitution (ie the entire condition) of a patient which should be treated, not just individual symptoms;
2 it works according to a 'law of similars' or 'like cures like', that is, the substance used to cure a condition is the same one that would cause that condition in healthy people; and
3 this second principle, together with the method of preparing the substances, are effective because they provide the energy to stimulate the body's own self-healing powers and immune system.

The following is a more technical explanation from Dr Eric:

Homoeopathy through the process of succussion (rhythmical agitation) with dilution and trituration (grinding) releases or imparts to the original substance a unique healing property analogous to a key. When there is proper alignment between the 'lock' (or the patient's symptoms and signs) and the 'key' (or remedy effects), then a specific healing response will occur. Modern pharmacological studies between drug receptors and blockers (for example Naloxone to block heroin overdose) work on a similar basis.

Homoeopathic remedies are prepared with purified water and alcohol. Unlike many pharmaceutical preparations they do not contain preservatives or additives other than alcohol. If a patient is extremely sensitive (I was when in severe relapse) the remedies can be made from purified water only, however their shelf life will be limited.

Homoeopathic remedies are also prepared in pillules of lactose which are given in a dose of 1 pillule dissolved in the mouth or dissolved in a glass of water and sipped over a period of time. According to Dr Eric, the lactose pillules are non-allergenic and can be taken even if suffering from diabetes as the dose is so small. As the remedy substance is of such a minute quantity contained in the base of water and alcohol or lactose they do not cause allergic reactions and side effects, nor do they cause harm to the body.

The dose for a baby or very small child is usually two drops on the tongue or for a very small baby, a few drops on the nipple before feeding. The adult dose is usually five drops. The general rule is that for acute illness the doses should initially be given at short intervals, say five to fifteen minutes. As improvement becomes apparent the intervals should be doubled with each dose, e.g. five minutes, ten minutes, twenty minutes, forty minutes etc. In the case of chronic illness the dose may be once, twice or three times per day until improvement occurs.

It is essential to understand that the remedies are not taken for a prolonged period. As soon as the symptoms disappear and you feel much better, the remedy should be stopped otherwise you may experience what is called a 'proving' and bring up further disease symptoms. Five to seven days would be about average, but sometimes the remedy is only required for a day or even a couple of doses. As soon as recovery is achieved, the remedy should be stopped because the symptoms have changed and that particular remedy is no longer required.

Unfortunately, homoeopathy is not accepted — and is even ridiculed — by many medical practitioners. My view is that 'if it works, why not try to understand it?'. One would think that according to the Hippocratic oath doctors would only be concerned with the well-being of their patients, so if a different form of medicine from the one to which they are accustomed works, why knock it? Acupuncture is a perfect example of this. Twenty years ago anyone who practised acupuncture was referred to as a 'quack' — now it is taught at some medical schools and the practice is available at some hospitals. Hopefully, more doctors will see the benefits of homoeopathic remedies which bring such blessed relief to patients and do not leave them suffering with terrible side effects. For myself I have nothing but praise and wonder for homoeopathy.

One criticism of homoeopathic remedies is that they work purely on a psychological basis but I believe this is a very misguided view. I can state quite categorically that not every remedy I have been given has worked in the same way; some have had a dramatic effect for the better, others have not made the slightest difference and a few have given me an adverse reaction. The adverse reaction is usually very short-lived, about one to three hours, is not serious or severe, and disappears. This is called a 'proving' or 'healing response'. Dr Eric usually advises me to leave it for 24 hours and take the remedy again. I have done this and started to improve almost immediately. Sometimes a remedy can bring on a 'healing crisis' when you will get worse before you start to get better. Do not panic — a good practitioner can usually provide a reason for this reaction but be sure to report it if it does happen. On the other hand, I have on occasions been completely bedridden and in total relapse, and after a couple of doses of a particular remedy I have felt a remarkable improvement and been able to get out of bed. If the remedy is correct the improvement is usually very quickly felt.

As there are so many homoeopathic remedies to cover such a variety of conditions, including your mental as well as you physical symptoms presenting at the time, it takes a very experienced practitioner to be able to sort out the correct remedy to match those symptoms. I cannot understand, therefore, why such a fascinating method of treatment, with no serious side effects, has for so long been ignored by the medical profession at large. Members of the Royal Family have used homoeopathy for years — the Queen takes a number of homoeopathic remedies with her when travelling. Of course, those forward-thinking and open-minded doctors who do dare to practise alternative medicine are often ridiculed by the majority of doctors, but are much sought after by patients who are sick and tired of being given something to relieve the symptoms, which often makes the patient much worse and creates other problems without effecting a cure. I can only recount my own experiences and say that homoeopathy has worked wonders for me.

When I started on the treatment, I could smell the rubbish coming out of my body in my urine, it had such a strong, strange smell. The first remedy I was given was Kali Carb (Carbonate of Potassium) and it was given to the 30th potency which is classed as 'average' (6th potency is low, 200th high and 1000 very high). The remedies are produced in the above potencies so that if it is suspected that someone is very sensitive, only the lowest (6th) potency is prescribed. I had a reaction (proving) to the influenza vaccine which was given to the 30th potency, but when given 1M (1000) potency, had no reaction at all. I did, however, seem to be protected from colds and flu even though I was exposed to them.

With an illness of such intensity and duration as ME/CFS,

it will take more than one remedy to make you better. With homoeopathic treatment the patient goes from one remedy to another as the symptoms change and, of course, with the varying symptoms of ME/CFS this is indeed a great advantage. Perseverance is required as it takes time — sometimes twelve months or more — to work the toxins out of the body and to stimulate the immune system to do its work. The remedies I have taken have been quoted in Dr Eric's report (see page 200) and there are a fair number of remedies but what suits me would not necessarily suit you, as each remedy has to match up perfectly with the symptoms presenting at the time and the type of personality you are.

On a quick count I would say I have been given over 30 remedies, some used only once and others used a number of times over the years. One of the most amazing remedies is the 'influenza and cold vaccine'. Just one dose (either 5 drops or 1 pillule) each month starting about March, then two doses per month in June and July, one dose per month till October and I have escaped colds and influenza. I have experimented on the family over the past four years and those who took the vaccine escaped or had a very mild cold while those who did not, succumbed. My husband was the last to be convinced, but last year he took them religiously and remained completely well whereas he had been quite ill the previous two years. He has already started them at the time of writing.

I must relate here a homoeopathic experience which should not be missed. It was around three months after my second relapse that I contracted a severe cold and tight cough. This necessitated a trip to Dr Eric. He was most perturbed at the sound of my chest and said I was on the verge of pneumonia. He gave me Arsenicum Alb, a homoeopathic remedy, and a prescription for penicillin; I was to keep up five drops of Ars. Alb. every four hours and if no better by morning to take the penicillin. I took my homoeopathic remedy and that night I ran a high fever. By morning the congestion had broken and I was well on my way to recovery. We had a real celebration as I had not been able to run a temperature since becoming ill. I did not need any antibiotics and I must say that since being introduced to homoeopathy and herbal remedies, except for one occasion which was disastrous, I have not required any other medicines.

I was listening to a farmer in New Zealand being interviewed on the ABC 'Country Wide' programme, explaining his homoeopathic treatment of sheep to prevent them from becoming fly-blown. He crushed the fly, mixed it homoeopathically and injected it into the mouth of the sheep. When asked how it worked, he said he didn't know, but it *did* work, so why question it? He runs a magnificent property in New Zealand and grows everything organically. He makes his own fertiliser from fish, and he treats all his animals homoeopathically. The results speak for themselves.

Homoeopathy for children

Children seem to respond extremely well to homoeopathy as it has safe and gentle remedies which apply to most childhood ailments without damaging the immune system.

One of the remarkable remedies which should be given just before and continued after innoculations is Thuja. This remedy helps to alleviate severe reactions to innoculations and is a most beneficial remedy to keep in the house. Two drops twice daily starting on the day before the innoculation and continued for three days afterwards helps the body to recover quickly.

Drugs should only be used as a last resort in babies and children. Their immune system takes at least two years to develop, so they should only be subjected to drugs, especially antibiotics which adversely affect the immune system, in the case of a life-threatening illness. That is where homoeopathy is so useful as the remedies act as an immune stimulant.

As you can see I have found great help in this form of medicine. I have enormous faith in it which must assist also, and I have taken the trouble to understand how it works in order to help myself. I cannot promise that homoeopathy and the other alternative remedies mentioned in this book will work as well for you — it is up to you also — but it is certainly something to investigate if all else has failed.

From my own experiences drugs have made me worse. Even before I contracted ME/CFS I could not tolerate them. An asprin made my stomach bloated and uncomfortable and 'the pill' caused me to black out. It has been a wonderful experience to find an alternative which has picked me up when I was down and eventually put me right back on my feet despite the severity of my relapses. In order to succeed, though, it is essential to find a highly qualified practitioner who is both medically qualified as well as qualified in alternative medicine. People who have such a combination of skills will be the medical practitioners of the future. My doctor is 20 years ahead of his time, and I thank the Lord that He put me into his care.

If I have stirred your interest in homoeopathy, a homoeopathic first aid kit can be purchased from Martin and Pleasance (through health food stores). This comes together with a pamphlet of remedies and symptoms which space prevents me from reprinting. A copy of the *Materia Medica* (the 'encyclopedia' of homoeopathy) is also available from them together with many other books on homoeopathy.

If you wish to find a homoeopathic doctor in your area, please consult the Directory (page 204).

Naturopathy and herbalism

There is some confusion these days between naturopathy and herbalism. In fact some people today who classify themselves as naturopaths understand and dispense herbal remedies almost exclusively. Technically, naturopathy advocates natural therapies such as fresh air and exercise instead of drugs or surgery. However, in our present-day society many people associate naturopaths with herbal remedies. Therefore, for the purposes of this book, we will classify naturopathy as embodying herbalism, acupuncture and other natural therapies other than drugs and surgery.

Homoeopathic and herbal remedies are similar but not the same. Homoeopathic remedies are made from the most minute amounts of substances like herbs, plants and venoms which are potentized as previously described. In other words they use the 'minimum' dose with the maximum effect, which is why they are particularly suitable for very sensitive and allergic people.

Herbal remedies are actual extracts from plants and herbs taken from the whole plant, the juice, the flowers, leaves or the root depending on the plant and its properties. For example, dandelion leaves are used to make 'tea' and the root is roasted and sold as 'dandelion coffee'. They are classified as a 'maximum' dose, so if you are particularly sensitive use a little caution. I personally have not had any adverse effects from herbal remedies, however I have only taken the 'concentrate'. Echinacea is dispensed in liquid form as a 'concentrate' or in a dried form in capsules. It can also be purchased in tablet form and as an ointment. Herbal remedies in tablet form are more likely to cause problems because of other additives.

I have used both homoeopathic and herbal remedies with great success as they both help to build up the immune system. So don't be downhearted if you cannot locate a homoeopathic doctor in your area. Try some of these herbal remedies which can be of great assistance. They are available from naturopaths, herbalists or health food stores.

Aloe Vera

Everyone should have an aloe vera plant in their garden or in a pot on their balcony. It looks like an ordinary green succulent plant with long fleshy leaves and small orange bell-like flowers. Cut off a piece of the leaf and inside there is a colourless gel which has remarkable healing qualities. It should be used externally for healing and can be taken internally for digestive problems. It is non-poisonous in small doses.

Arnica

This is the complete opposite of calendula. It is *never* used on broken skin, but has a marvellous effect on bruises and sprains and will relieve muscle and rheumatic pain. The homoeopathic form (5 drops) can be given to relieve muscle aches and pains, and one dose given to a child after a fall will reduce shock and bruising. Arnica is usually only available from health food stores in ointment form. (Homoeopathic arnica is one of the remedies in the First Aid Kit available from Martin and Pleasance, see Directory page 204).

Calendula

This is a remarkable extract from the calendula marigold and has incredible healing powers on any cuts or wounds, particularly ulcers and abscesses. When my cat developed an abscess after a fight, I kept applying drops of calendula extract onto his paw and within five days it was completely healed. I recently sent a bottle to a friend of mine for her mouth ulcers. She noted that I recommended it for cuts and wounds so decided to try it on her hands which had severe cracks and eruptions because of a detergent allergy. She used it for one day and rang me dumbfounded because her hands were healing up before her eyes. She said 'What is in it? It is miraculous!' It can be purchased in ointment form, but I prefer the concentrate (also referred to as 'mother tincture')

While using a lanoline based calendula ointment I developed sores on my lips which defied diagnosis. Pathology tests were negative. In the end I attributed it to the probable pesticide residue in the lanoline. In desperation I ended up making my own lip salve from natural oils. (See page 173 for the recipe.)

Chamomile

Chamomile has long been known as one of the most important medicinal plants. It is anti-inflammatory and inhibits bacterial growth. It is delicious as a tea and can even be given to small babies for wind and colic. It is used extensively in Europe for all gastric upsets.

Chelidonium

A liver remedy. Dr Eric dispenses this in herbal concentrate form to drain the liver. As most ME/CFS patients seem to have liver problems this is a wonderful remedy for clearing the liver of toxins.

Cretaegus

Excellent remedy for high blood pressure and irregularity of the heart. I recently had a very accelerated pulse rate and this was the prescribed remedy. It worked.

Dandelion

The root can be readily purchased and makes a delicious nutty coffee which is good for the liver and recommended for hepatitis. Tea made from the leaves is excellent as a diuretic and helpful in urinary and kidney problems. Both are availble from health food stores.

Echinacea

A remarkable remedy for improving the immune system. It has a beneficial effect on the blood count (increases the white cells) and septic conditions generally. It should be given after severe illness (except where there is a problem with the white blood cell count as in leukemia) especially if tiredness persists. It is an ideal remedy for those with ME/CFS. I have tried and proven it and so has my family. It is excellent for glandular fever.

Garlic

Garlic is nature's own antibiotic, antiseptic and expectorant for inducing sweating, and as an agent for reducing blood pressure. Garlic is recommended in the treatment of thrush as it has anti-fungal properties. It has also been used in the treatment of high cholesterol, hardening of the arteries and prevention of colds.

Horseradish

This is an effective remedy for allergies which cause hay fever or mild asthma. Procurable in tablets and drops from health food stores.

Phytolacca

Phytolacca is often given in conjunction with echinacea. It is prominently a glandular remedy and the two remedies are very beneficial during breastfeeding. It is beneficial to ME/CFS patients with glandular problems. This is a tried and proven remedy of my family. It can be poisonous if the maximum of 10 drops per day of the tincture is exceeded. Both Echinacea and Phytolacca work through their mitogens which amplify the immune response.

Slippery elm

The inner bark of the elm may be used to great advantage. This remedy is excellent for any inflammation of the gastro-intestinal tract. It soothes inflamed tissue. It should be taken when any gastric or digestive upset overtakes you, including diarrhoea. It can be purchased in powder or tablet form and as a food supplement (Healtheries) for invalids at health food stores.

As a general rule herbal remedies in 'concentrate form' are dispensed by naturopaths/herbalists. Most health food stores keep only tablets, capsules, ointments and lotions. For further product information see chapter 10.

The Bach Flower remedies

Let not the simplicity of this method deter you from its use, for you will find the further your researches advance, the greater you will realise the simplicity of all Creation.

Take no notice of the disease; think only of the outlook on life of the one in distress.

Final and complete healing will come from within, from the Soul itself, which by His beneficence radiates harmony throughout the personality when allowed to do so.

The above are quotes from Dr Edward Bach MBBS, MRCS, LRCP, DPH a great physician who practised for many years as a Harley Street consultant and bacteriologist. He practised homoeopathy and is responsible for the seven oral vaccines, named Seven Bach Nosodes which are used successfully today. In 1930 he gave up his practice to seek healing from the plant world. His remedies are prescribed not for the physical complaint, but rather for the sufferer's state of mind. His philosophy was that an inharmonious state of mind hinders the recovery of health.

The following chart of Dr Bach's remedies has been compiled by Martin and Pleasance, the Australian distributors of the Bach Flower Remedies and they are available either directly from them or through your health food stores. They are absolutely harmless and can be used on the elderly, babies, animals and plants.

Guide to Bach Flower Remedies

When choosing a remedy from the chart, locate the most outstanding negative aspect. Other remedies can be chosen to support this and guide toward a positive mental outlook.

Uncertainty

unsure of self repeatedly seeks advice from others	indecision and hesitancy inbalance	depression from known cause pessimism and easily discouraged	depression of long duration utter despondency	inability to cope with daily tasks lack of strength
Cerato	Scleranthus	Gentian	Gorse	Hornbeam

Fear

extreme fear and panic terror	fear of known things eg. heights, poverty etc.	desperate and suicidal fears own actions in desperation	vague fears of unknown origin anxiety and apprehension	excessive fear for others irrational anxieties
Rock Rose	Mimulus	Cherry Plum	Aspen	Red Chestnut

Loneliness   Insufficient

pride and aloofness desire to be alone	impatience and irritability	over concern with self but dislike being alone	dreams of the future inattention	nostalgia absorbed in memories of the past
Water Violet	Impatiens	Heather	Clematis	Honeysuckle

Despondency and Despair

feels inferior expectation of failure	feeling of guilt and self-doubt	overwhelmed by responsibilities and feelings of inadequacy	mental anguish having reached limits of endurance	for shock, physical, mental or emotional
Larch	Pine	Elm	Sweet Chestnut	Star of Bethlehem

Place 2 drops of the chosen remedies either directly onto the tongue or dilute in a little water or fruit juice. Take at least 4 times daily or more often when necessary. Store in a cool, dark place.

	Oversensitivity			
unsure of path in life lack of knowing what to do	mental worry and torture but appear cheerful	easily influenced and exploited by others	at times of great change sensitivity to outside influences	jealously and suspicion feelings of revenge
Wild Oat	*Agrimony*	*Centaury*	*Walnut*	*Holly*

Overcare For Others Welfare				
self-indulgent and self-pity	desire to influence others	desire to dominate others ruthless and inflexible	criticism and intolerance judgemental attitude	self denial and martyrdom
Chicory	*Vervain*	*Vine*	*Beech*	*Rockwater*

Interest in Present Circumstances				
apathy and resignation	complete physical and mental exhaustion	persistent worrying thoughts	deep gloom and depression from unknown cause	failure to learn from past experiences repeats the same mistakes
Wild Rose	*Olive*	*White Chestnut*	*Mustard*	*Chestnut Bud*

bitterness, resentment and blaming others for own mistakes	effects of endurance when under pressure	self condemnation over concentration on trivia	**Rescue Remedy** *A combination of five Bach flower remedies. These are Star of Bethlehem, Rock Rose, Impatiens, Clematis and Cherry Plum.*
Willow	*Oak*	*Crab Apple*	*These are chosen to meet most emergencies or accidents and help restore balance in stressful situations.*

Having considered these alternative remedies, may I recommend a book by Dr David Collison, Clinical Ecologist *Why Do I Feel So Awful?* which points out that medical science can, on many occasions, make the patient worse rather than better. He is critical of the many drugs freely dispensed which can have very serious side effects of which the patient is not made aware.

This is not in any way denegrating medical science which has discovered miracle cures and made remarkable progress in the fields of surgery and medical technology, but it does point to a need for alternative, natural, safe remedies which do not have serious side effects or damage the body. Therefore, in my humble opinion, there is a place for homoeopathy, herbalism, acupuncture, chiropractic and osteopathy, nutrition and other natural therapies when practised by skilled and qualified persons and it is a pity that they are so unacceptable to the medical profession at large.

The Therapeutic Goods Act 1989 which was passed last year, and the regulations relating thereto which are currently (May 1990) under discussion in the Senate, unless revised, will severely restrict the availability of homoeopathic and herbal remedies. Whilst we need to be protected from unqualified practitioners and from contaminated remedies and therapeutic aids, chiropractors and osteopaths, although both registered and recognised practitioners, are not exempt from the Act. Physiotherapists are exempt. Natural therapists such as naturopaths, herbalists, homoeopaths, acupuncturists, although qualified, are not recognised at all under the Act but are referred to as members of the public. We all have a right to freedom of choice. Please all speak up for our right of choice by writing to The Hon. Peter Staples, Minister for Housing and Aged Care, to Dr Robert Woods, Shadow Minister for Health and Senator John Coulter, Parliament House, Canberra, to ensure that the remedies which are presently available from our natural therapists and health food stores will continue to be so available.

8   Vitamins, Minerals and Diet

Vitamins

If the lawn is fertilised with superphosphate or sulphate of ammonia it will grow very quickly and look extremely green. However, in the process of such fast growth, it is highly likely that the grass will not contain all the nutrients it would have 'taken up' if it had been fertilised naturally.

It has been found that organically grown plants contain more protein, minerals and sugar than those grown with a quick growth, artificial fertiliser. Although it seems a contradiction in terms, it has been found that the higher sugar content of the organically grown plant makes it more resistant to pests. I have found that seaweed is a wonderful fertiliser, especially for the vegetables, and by planting herbs amongst the garden, I have not been greatly troubled by pests. I understand that the American Indians used to plant a fish with each seed of corn — fish is wonderful fertiliser also. (They also planted three seeds — one for the birds, one for the insects and one for themselves. Maybe we could learn a lesson from them.)

It seems that with our modern-day, force-grown, sprayed and processed food, and the constant exposure to toxins, we need vitamin and mineral supplements in order to stay well. Those who are lucky enough to be able to grow or buy organically grown vegetables, fruit and meat, together with organically grown grains and naturally dried fruits, should be able to provide themselves with a healthy diet.

Whatever diet is followed, tailored to your own specific requirements and food allergies, it is important to note that cooking destroys many vitamins, minerals and enzymes. Therefore uncooked fresh fruit and vegetables should constitute a major part of our daily diet. Many enzymes, destroyed by cooking, are necessary for proper digestion of that particular food. If we look at nature, and the foods provided for us, it is obvious that we should be eating them as nature intended in order to derive the most benefit from them.

Similarly pasteurising our milk may kill the bacteria, but it also kills essential enzymes which enable it to be digested properly. Obviously our methods of mass production, although convenient and eliminating bacteria, have created problems of their own.

(By the way, Dr Eric does not advocate introducing cow's milk to children until they are twelve months old to avoid milk sensitisation.)

A point to remember, also, is that mass production, importation and transportation, cold storage and refrigeration provide us with an all-year-round supply of many fruits and vegetables which used to be seasonal. Therefore people tend to eat the same foods day after day. This is most unnatural. It is much better to eat foods in season and to give the body a rest from them between seasons. Freshly picked, organically grown, unrefrigerated fruit and vegetables eaten raw will provide the maximum of essential vitamins and minerals to keep us healthy.

Most ME/CFS sufferers benefit from vitamin supplements, especially the B Group, including biotin, but again you will have to work out your own programme. Vitamins A, C and

E act as anti-oxidants which assist in eliminating toxins from the body. L-Cysteine, a natural amino acid, is also recommended in this regard. Do not forget that cod liver oil is a natural source of Vitamins A and D so be careful not to overdose if you are already taking vitamin supplements. The recommended dosage of Vitamin A is 5000 iu (international units) per day. All vitamins should be taken with medical supervision because, if you are extremely sensitive, even the tablet fillers may upset you . 'CAL C' which contains a calcium buffer is recommended, especially as it will cause the least upset to your stomach. I have found 'FAB' (natural iron plus B group vitamins) very helpful at various times, as well as Formula 3 'Vita Glow' (zinc, magnesium, B6 and dolomite).

Blackmores 'Naturetime' is a high potency vitamin and mineral preparation and I have found this beneficial too, especially when I have been feeling fatigued. Do not take several preparations at the same time — read the labels and make sure you do not 'double up'. Overdosing on anything can be very dangerous which is why it is better to consult an expert when taking vitamin and mineral therapy. Listen to your body to see if you feel 'better' or 'worse' (if you have any adverse reaction of course discontinue the therapy). However do give vitamin therapy time to help you — it sometimes takes a few weeks.

A friend of mine was diagnosed as being deficient in zinc. She was put on a fairly high dosage of zinc in a combination vitamin and mineral formulation for three weeks. She improved considerably and put on weight. Just before the end of the three week period she found she was getting a metallic taste in her mouth after taking the tablet. Her body was possibly giving her the message that she no longer required the high dosage. I am just quoting this as an example of the fact that we must not blindly take any medication, vitamins or minerals if our body is telling us it is not happy.

I am setting out here a brief guide to the vitamins which occur naturally in our foods, so that you do not overdose on any one food, but keep a balanced approach to your eating habits. In my view, this applies to the whole of life — moderation in all things!

Vitamin A

Helps maintain skin, eyes, urinary tract, and linings of the nervous, respiratory and digestive systems. Needed for normal growth of bones and teeth, and for good night vision.

Foods which contain Vitamin A/Betacarotene: sweet potatoes, milk, liver, fish liver oils, eggs, butter, green and yellow vegetables.

Vitamin B1 (Thiamin)

Needed for carbohydrate metabolism and release of energy from food. Helps heart and nervous system function properly.

Foods which contain Vitamin B1: yeast, meat, wholegrain cereals, nuts, soybeans, peas, potatoes, most vegetables.

Vitamin B2 (Riboflavin)

Helps body cells use oxygen. Promotes tissue repair and healthy skin.

Foods which contain Vitamin B2: milk, cheese, liver, heart, fish, poultry.

Niacin

Essential for cell metabolism and absorption of carbohydrates. Helps maintain healthy skin. Relieves depression and tiredness.

Foods which contain Niacin: liver, yeast, lean meat.

Vitamin B6

Needed for healthy teeth and gums, blood vessels, nervous system, and red blood cells.

Foods which contain Vitamin B6: yeast, whole-grain cereals, meat, wheatgerm, most vegetables.

Vitamin B12

Essential for proper development of red blood cells. Helps proper function of nervous system.

Foods which contain B12: eggs, meat, milk, milk products.

Biotin

Needed for healthy circulatory system and for maintaining healthy skin.

Foods which contain Biotin: eggs, liver, kidney, most fresh vegetables.

Folic Acid

Needed for production of red blood cells.

Foods which contain Folic Acid: green leafy vegetables, yeast, meat.

Vitamin C (Ascorbic Acid)

Essential for sound bones and teeth. Needed for tissue metabolism and wound healing.

Foods which contain Vitamin C: citrus fruits, tomatoes, raw cabbage, potatoes, strawberries, cantaloupe.

Vitamin D

Essential for calcium and phosphorous metabolism.

Foods which contain Vitamin D: fish liver oils, fortified milk, eggs, tuna, salmon. Sunlight activates Vitamin D in the skin.

Vitamin E

Helps maintain heart and skeletal muscles, and may help maintain reproductive system.

Foods which contain Vitamin E: wholegrain cereals, lettuce, cold pressed vegetable oils.

Vitamin K

Needed for normal blood clotting.

Foods which contain Vitamin K: leafy vegetables, buck-wheat. Vitamin K is made by intestinal bacteria.

Minerals

Minerals are crucial to our well-being. They are more important than vitamins, and whereas vitamins constitute less than 1 per cent of our body weight, minerals constitute 5 per cent. It is important to realise that vitamins are often dependent on minerals for their absorption and biochemical functions, so it is necessary that we eat a balanced diet of nutritional foods.

Plants take their minerals from the rocks, soil and water, and animals eat the plants. Just as the quality of our food and its mineral content is essential to our well-being, the quality of pastures and grains are essential to the well-being of the farm animals and birds which provide most of us with our meat. The quality of our rivers and oceans will determine the quality of our fish and seafood. Naturally grown, unpolluted food is the answer.

Although I would in no way profess to be an expert, I have listed below the minerals, trace elements and their sources to give you a guide to our nutritional needs, and to encourage you to read books written by experts on the subject (see pages 103 & 104). All mineral supplements should be taken with the approval, and under the direction, of your practitioner, as too much of one particular mineral could affect the absorption of another.

Mineral	Food source
Calcium	Sardines, soy milk, milk products, sesame seeds, molasses, nuts, soy products
Magnesium	Meat, fish, poultry, nuts, bran, milk, honey, eggs, green vegetables, brewer's yeast, brown rice
Phosphorus	Milk, meat, eggs, grains, yellow cheeses

Potassium	Meat, fish, bananas, vegetables, dates, figs, peaches
Sodium	Salt, celery, milk and cheese
Sulphur	Green vegetables and dates

Bone meal is a source of calcium and phosphorus.
Dolomite is a source of magnesium and calcium.
Kelp is a source of choline, sodium and sulphur.
Molasses is a source of potassium.

Trace element	Food source
Chromium	Yeast, liver, brewer's yeast, wholegrains, liver, cheese, molasses and rye
Copper	Seafood, legumes, liver and nuts
Cobalt	Most foods
Iron	Liver, meat, brewer's yeast and eggs
Iodine	Seafood and kelp
Manganese	Wheat germ, seeds, legumes, buckwheat, nuts
Molybdenium	Lentils and most foods
Selenium	Whole wheat, garlic. Generally speaking Australia is deficient in selenium.
Zinc	Corn, oysters, carrots, ginger, mushrooms, sunflower seeds.

Remember that soaking vegetables in water can cause the mineral content to be partially lost. Try steaming to retain goodness. Of course, vegetables and fruit eaten raw will provide the maximum of vitamins and minerals.

Minerals and their interaction with vitamins and other minerals are not as yet fully understood, however much evidence is coming forth to place great importance on them as an essential ingredient to our well-being. I would refer you to the following books which are fascinating and useful.

Your Health Vitamins and Minerals, Russell Frank Atkinson, 1982.

Your Personal Health Programme, Dr Jeffrey Bland, 1984.

(See Directory for organically-grown vegetables, fruit and meat. Page 211)

A DIFFERENT APPROACH TO DIET — THE HAY SYSTEM

I have tried the following system and found it kind to the digestion. It presents a different approach and may assist in alleviating problems which many experience with digestion. The theory of this system — the Hay system — of eating is that by combining certain foods, and not others, it seems to make the job easier for the digestive juices. It is a most thought provoking theory and it's certainly worth considering, particularly if you are experiencing such effects as indigestion, discomfort, bloating, loose motions. You will not put on weight — in fact you may lose some and you may need to eat potatoes (being an alkaline starch) between meals, or even have more frequent meals. I have friends who use the diet during the week, and then 'sin' during the weekend. They were suffering Post Viral Fatigue following a severe virus, and found the diet, together with plenty of rest, very helpful in the rehabilitation process.

The Hay System — A Brief Summary

The diet was developed by Dr William Howard Hay, Pennsylvania, USA, in the 1930s, based on sound and proven physiological principles (i.e. different enzymes are required to break up and digest proteins and carbohydrates; drinking with meals dilutes gastric acids, thereby making the job of digestion less effective etc.)

Following the Hay System will shed unneccessary weight, allow far greater absorption of all vitamins and minerals in our food and lead generally to better health and well-being.

Five important rules

1   Starches and sugars (carbohydrates) should not be eaten with proteins and acid fruit at the same meal.
2   Vegetables, salads and fruits should form the major part of the diet.
3   Proteins, starches and fats should be eaten in small quantities.
4   Only wholegrain and unprocessed starches should be used, and all refined, processed foods should be taboo — in particular, white flour and sugar and all foods made with them, and highly processed fats such as margarine.
5   An interval of at least four to four and a half hours should elapse before eating meals of different character.

Brief explanation

Proteins are concentrated (20 per cent or more) animal proteins such as meat, fish, cheese, poultry.

Carbohydrates are concentrated (20 per cent or more) starches such as grains, bread and cereals, potatoes; and sugars.

Although meat does contain carbohydrates this is in the form of glycogen which requires little if any digestion and therefore does not interfere with the digestion of proteins.

Similarily, the protein content in grains is incomplete in character and therefore does not interfere with the conditions necessary for starch digestion.

Exception to the rules: mature or dried legumes (peas, beans, lentils, peanuts) are incompatible with one another (except when sprouted). Unless you have built up a tolerance to these over many years they should be left alone.

COMPATIBLE FOODS

Columns I and III are incompatible

can be combined   can be combined

I	II	III
For Protein meals	*Neutral Foods* can be combined with either Col. I or Col. III	*For Starch meals*

PROTEINS	**NUTS**	**CEREALS**
Meat of all kinds: Beef, lamb, pork, venison	All except peanuts	Wholegrain: Wheat barley, maize (corn), oats, millet rice (brown, unpolished), rye
Poultry: Chicken, duck, goose, turkey Game: Pheasant, patridge, grouse, hare	FATS Butter Cream Egg yolks Olive oil (virgin)	Bread 100% wholewheat Flour 100% or 85% Oatmeal — medium
Fish of all kinds including shellfish	Sunflower seed oil Sesame seed oil (cold pressed)	
Eggs Cheese Milk (combines best with fruit and should not be served at a meat meal) Yogurt		

FRUITS	**VEGETABLES**	**SWEET FRUITS**
Apples Apricots (Fresh)	All green and root (dried)	Bananas — ripe vegetables except potatoes Dates
Blackberries Blueberries Cherries Currants (black, red or white if ripe) Gooseberries (if ripe) Grapefruit	Jerusalem artichokes Asparagus Aubergines (Eggplants) Beans (all fresh green beans) Beetroot Broccoli	Figs (fresh & dried) Grapes — extra sweet Papaya if *very* ripe Pears if *very* sweet and ripe Currants Raisins

Columns I and III are incompatible

can be combined   can be combined

I	II	III
FRUITS	**VEGETABLES**	**SWEET FRUITS**
Grapes	Brussels sprouts	Sultanas
Kiwis	Cabbage	
Lemons	Carrots	**VEGETABLES**
Limes	Cauliflower	
Loganberries	Celery	Potatoes
Mangoes	Celeriac	Jerusalem artichokes
Melons (best eaten	Courgettes (zucchini)	
alone as a fruit meal)	Kohlrabi	**MILK & YOGURT**
Nectarines	Leeks	
Oranges	Marrow (squash)	only in moderation
Papayas	Mushrooms	
Pears	Onions	
Pineapples	Parsnips	
Prunes (or occasional	Peas	
use)	Spinach	
Raspberries	Swedes	
Satsumas	Turnips	
Strawberries		
Tangerines		
N.B. plums and cranberries		
are *not* recommended		

I	II	III
SALAD DRESSINGS	**SALAD VEGETABLES**	**SALAD DRESSINGS**
French dressing made	Avocados	Sweet or soured cream
with oil and lemon	Chicory (endive)	Olive oil or cold
juice or apple cider	Corn salad	pressed seed oils
vinegar	Cucumber	Fresh tomato juice with oil
Cream dressing	Endive (chicory)	and seasoning
Mayonnaise (homemade)	Fennel	
	Garlic	
	Lettuce	
	Mustard & cress	
	Peppers, red and green	
	Radishes	

Columns I and III are incompatible

can be combined   can be combined

I	II	III
SALAD DRESSINGS	**SALAD VEGETABLES**	**SALAD DRESSINGS**

SALAD VEGETABLES

Spring onions (scallions)
Sprouted legumes
Sprouted seeds
Tomatoes (uncooked)
Watercress

HERBS & FLAVOURINGS

Chives
Mint
Parsley
Sage
Tarragon
Thyme
Grated lemon rind
Grated orange rind

SEEDS

Sunflower
Sesame
Pumpkin

BRAN

Wheat or oat bran
Wheatgerm

SUGAR	**SUGAR SUBSTITUTES**	**SUGAR SUBSTITUTES**
Diluted frozen orange juice	Raisins and raisin juice Honey	Barbados sugar Honey — in strict moderation
FOR VEGETARIANS (but not recommended)	Maple syrup	
Legumes Lentils Soya beans		

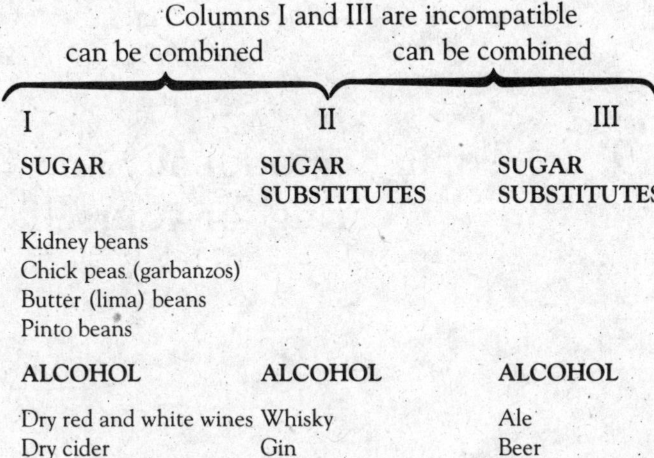

Note: A combination of foods from columns I & II constitutes a protein meal. A combination of foods from columns II & III constitutes a starch meal. Foods in columns I & III should not be eaten at the same meal.

I am extremely grateful to Thorsons Publishing Group Ltd, UK, for allowing me to republish the Hay system of eating as set out in *Food Combining for health* by Doris Grant and Jean Joice. The book contains menus and recipes as well and should be read in total if you intend to follow this diet.

9   Coping emotionally and caring for yourself

Listening to our bodies

In retrospect my body was giving me messages for many years that certain chemicals were affecting me. Strong-smelling substances such as bleach, paints and wood stains would cause me to lose my sense of smell and make my nose bleed. I also suffered from pustules in my nostrils, bloodshot sore eyes, seemed to have continual catarrh and eventually became very short of breath. I did not pay any attention at the time, but I realise now I would quite often get a sore throat which did not develop into a throat infection or cold. I would often feel very thirsty. I noticed that I did not like the smell of certain substances, particularly petrol and kerosene. This can indicate also, Leonie tells me, a deficiency in zinc. If only I had listened to my body I would not have absorbed so much and would not have done myself so much damage. The lesson to be learned is — *if a smell offends you — avoid it.* This includes many household cleaners, perfumes and cosmetics, not just substances we more typically think of as being 'chemical'. (Unfortunately not everyone has such a keen sense of smell. I have one friend, totally invalided with ME/CFS, who has lost her sense of smell completely.

Consequently she has great difficulty avoiding toxins which send her into relapse.)

Often I would come home from the shops and feel exhausted although I had not overexerted myself. It took some time to realise that in shopping centres I was being exposed to toxic fumes emanating from the shopping environment or the products sold there, so that the fatigue I felt was not necessarily caused by exertion. Take a note, when out and about, of just how much pollution is evident by way of petrol and exhaust fumes, cigarette smoke, fumes from products, hairdressing salons, perfumes, newly decorated premises, clothing shops and many more. You will become much more aware of them and so minimise your exposure.

When in severe relapse, which on every occasion has been after exposure to toxic chemicals, I experienced a cold burning (like hot ice) or pins and needles, under the skin and trembling of the legs as though I had a motor running in them. They felt very 'restless' at this stage and I had difficulty relaxing them in bed and of course difficulty in sleeping. The burning under the skin occurred after I had been exposed to petrochemicals and pesticides, and especially phenol.

My body was giving me another message. When I inhaled certain toxic chemicals I would get a headache, or would become very agitated and vague and was completely unable to organise myself. As I had always been an excellent organiser, this was very difficult to accept.

Your feelings about food can also give you a clue about substances which trigger your illness. Do you *love* to eat a certain food, or *hate* another? If so, the chances are you are highly intolerant of or allergic to both. That is the body giving you a message, so avoid those foods.

It is interesting to note here that the taste and smell of both penicillin and flagyl were so abhorrent to me that I had great difficulty taking them. Both these drugs contributed to my illness. Although there are times when antibiotics are a wonderful lifesaver, on many occasions I should have listened more to my body's reaction.

My body was giving me messages years ago to slow down. I was getting tension headaches and terrible tightness in the neck and shoulders. At times my digestive system would refuse to work and I would have to take a week's holiday to get myself back to normal.

Of course I was trying to do too much. I should have taken stock of my life, sorted out what was really important, and left the rest. Apart from a house and children, I was involved in amateur musicals, making my own costumes and sewing clothes for myself and my daughter, so when I think back I would have had to be a superwoman to keep up the pace. It was just one long rush and I would push and push, ignoring tiredness. It is no wonder I eventually succumbed to illness, this frantic pace would surely have had yet another detrimental effect on my immune system. We must learn to recognise the fact that we are tired and need rest. We cannot push our bodies forever, otherwise we put them into a very stressful state where the adrenal glands are working overtime and so giving our bodies a continual flow of adrenalin which nature never intended. Take heed, then, and learn to relax.

If you find yourself getting hyped-up, just slow all your movements down and do things very slowly (as in slow motion). This has a very calming effect. You must mentally slow down, too, and take the attitude that, whatever the cause of the panic, it is not the end of the world. If you are running late, so what? If an accident has occurred, even though it may be serious, concentrate on staying calm because you will achieve much more in this frame of mind. You will think more clearly, and act so much more efficiently. So, no matter what happens, if the children make a complete mess, is it really so terrible? A positive, calm attitude of mind can really work wonders on the way our body functions.

I used to worry about so many unnecessary things which were quite unimportant, really. I think I have created a far happier home where everyone feels completely relaxed as a result of my change of attitude. A house that looks like a picture out of *House and Garden* is no longer my idea of home. Recognise these factors and that rest and relaxation are a very important part of *everyday* life. Techniques to encourage a state of relaxation are discussed later in this chapter.

Without becoming a hypochondriac, take note of your bowel movements. If they are not normal (i.e. if they are loose, foamy, pale, very dark, constipated etc.) this can indicate a food allergy, digestive upset or even candida/thrush attacking the intestines and bowel. (Candida/thrush is discussed later in this chapter.) Take a note of what you have eaten that day, then by way of elimination try to find the culprit(s). Procedures for testing by way of elimination can be found in Dr Mackarness's book *Chemical Victims*. This excellent book is very inexpensive and offers a wealth of information.

A good example of 'listening to my body' occurred recently. I seemed to constantly have loose foamy motions. Since I discovered 'Demeter' organically-grown rolled oats, I had been eating them regularly — nearly every morning, in fact, with stewed apples. The taste is superb and reminds me of the oats we used to eat when I was a child. However, I had apparently overdone my consumption of oats and as soon as I stopped eating them my motions returned to normal. I am giving my body a chance to recover for a few weeks and will then introduce them slowly and in *moderation*.

You should also pay attention to your pulse rate which may rise after you eat a food to which you are intolerant or after you have come in contact with any chemical which disagrees with you. You may even experience palpitations. In *Chemical Victims* Dr Mackarness sets out a section on chemical testing procedures also. These are provocation tests. However, be careful not to expose yourself to a large dose of fumes which you know could cause relapse. It is interesting to note that Dr Mackarness found that some patients with allergies to various foods, including wheat and chicken, did not have the same allergic reaction when given organically-grown foods.

I have a friend who has constant trouble with palpitations and panic attacks. She cannot eat a large meal without getting palpitations, and certain food will trigger them off. However, with perseverance she has managed to find the foods which were causing the problem. In her case it was bread additives and preservatives. She found that breads baked with organically-grown grains, without additives, seemed to be far more satisfactory.

Take note, also, of your basic body rhythms. Should changes occur in temperature, menstrual cycle or sleep patterns, something may be amiss, so visit your medical practitioner before a severe problem develops.

In short, it is important to listen to our bodies. It is constantly giving us clues as to the foods and substances it does not like by way of odour reaction, sinus, catarrh, diarrhoea, constipation, foamy stools, sore nose, sore throat, asthma, shortness of breath, bleeding nose, sore and/or watery eyes, stomach-ache, bloated stomach, indigestion, heartburn, palpitations, accelerated pulse rate, skin eruptions or dermatitis, hay fever, arthritis, headache, vertigo, disorientation, itching and dandruff or hair problems.

Listen to the messages and you will find that by taking a little care and time, your health will improve tremendously.

Understanding illness

When I first became aware that I had a severe long-term illness I was devastated. It was so foreign to me not to 'bounce back', as I had always done in the past, that I found it very difficult to accept and come to terms with the situation. I had always 'run at a million miles an hour' and had the reputation of being able to do in one week what it took most other people one month to do. I enjoyed life and achievement and hated 'wasting time'. I had many hobbies and was always dreaming up new avenues to conquer, besides being devoted to my family. I know I went into shock for some weeks and was very angry. I soon realised that this was not going to achieve anything, so I decided to make my illness work for me.

There had been times previously when I longed to have nothing to do and here I was unable to do anything! I used to dream of not having to get up early each morning, and here I was experiencing such luxury. I now had time to listen to music and to the radio which is such a good educator. I had always loved reading, but never had enough time, so when my eyes were working, I read and read. I would take time to lie outside and watch the sky and the trees and the birds and be at peace with nature, something I'd rarely had time to do. I took time to think about my family, all their needs and the wonderful times we had spent together when the children were young. I made plans for what I would like to do when I was well *for I was going to get well*, that I determined.

How often have you said I'm too busy now, tell me later,' to your children, partner or friends? Take some of your 'body resting time' to talk to your children and friends, in small doses, though, to avoid fatigue. When you are feeling well enough, take the time to play with them whatever games they choose whether it's snakes and ladders, draughts, jigsaw puzzles, Scrabble, or Trivial Pursuit. You now have *time* to talk to your family and friends in small doses. Just think, if you had not become sick, so necessitating rest, you would not have had the time to share these quiet activities. (It was during this period that our telephone bill went through the roof!) Even just lying quietly on the bed with a child or partner can give you both comfort and reassurance.

Mentally plan what you can do when you are better. I suppose I should say here 'Tape your thoughts, plan a book', but I must be honest and admit that I did not give it a thought.

Plan a redecorating scheme, mentally change the furniture around, plan a new garden or a new outfit particularly if you are good with the needle. If you are strong enough, drawing, knitting (not for too long, though), tapestry, embroidery or other handicrafts are very therapeutic. At one stage I managed to do some china painting.

I know this is very easy to say, for there may be times when you feel too ill to care what happens. These are times you should curl up into your little shell and opt out. Do not feel guilty — it is part of the recovery process.

Leonie was wonderful during my times of immobilisation for she lent me many books on medicine, especially on homoeopathy. I was fascinated by this method of treatment, as it really worked, and I decided that I could help myself much more if I understood its principles. There is no doubt that this has proven to be so, to the extent that I can now choose the right remedy for myself and others on many occasions. With practice you do become proficient enough to prescribe for many minor ailments. At the end of this book I have listed books on homoeopathy to read if I have fired your curiosity. *The Magic of the Minimum Dose* by Dr Dorothy Shepherd was the first book I read as it is totally uncomplicated. Although first published in 1938 and subseqently revised, it is as applicable today as it was then, given that homoeopathy has not changed in the last 100 years. Dr Eric runs classes for parents, teaching them the basic principles of this medicine so that they can care for their families quickly and easily during non-serious illnesses. How practical! I sometimes wish I had medical qualifications so that I could study to become a homoeopath myself.

Many of us seem to take 'living' for granted until we are immobilised for some time. To appreciate being alive is something we easily forget. We are always planning for tomorrow instead of living, to the fullest of our ability, today. We do not have to rush around to *live* — this is something I have learned through my experience, and I take time out of each day to relax and enjoy what I have, and what I can do. If you have ever watched *Monkey* on TV you may have heard his lesson: 'Why do we *want* so much, when we *need* so little?' That quote has stuck in my mind.

I found it amazing how much can be learned about yourself and others when you are struck down. I became far more considerate and sympathetic to the needs of others and I realised that all the money in the world could not buy health and happiness, for without health you cannot live life to its absolute fullest. However, I did appreciate so very much those who cared for me even when I was at my lowest. This takes a very understanding partner and I think that the partner is often the one who needs counselling rather than the patient.

Children can become irritable when a parent is out of action because in their eyes the world appears to have collapsed around them. I have deep sympathy and understanding for sick people with young children. I don't think we can expect the children to understand, but I do think we can expect them to be kind. And it is remarkable how often we, as parents, take all the responsibility for our children although they can and do respond if the ball is thrown into their court. The most important element in these circumstances is good communication and approaching the problem by making them feel they are helping to solve it. When I asked my children, 'How do you think we should do this, or that, or how can we make life at home better for all concerned?' I was surprised at some of their suggestions. Encouragement and making them feel important is the key to success here rather than complaints and criticism.

Except for my daughter (who had been sick herself and was always most caring and kind — she is a very special daughter) the other children, four boys, were all teenagers when I became ill. It has taken time for them to understand fully the implications of ME/CFS but even though they may not have done too much housewise (my husband was so capable in this regard) they would pop in to have a word with me, to see how I was feeling. It was all I needed to know that I had to rehabilitate myself, for I was well loved.

One of the coincidences of life occurred just before my third severe relapse. I had always been interested in politics and had joined a political party some ten years previously. As I was no longer working, I decided to join the party's women's committee and accordingly went to a meeting in the city. Although I had been diagnosed as having ME/CFS by Dr Eric I had interpreted it as a type of encephalitis and had not really bothered to find out what it meant or what it was all about, as under his treatment and my study of homoeopathy I had twice gone through the process of recovery. During the course of this meeting, a community service booklet was handed around and as I flicked through the pages my eye caught a page which said 'Are you constantly fatigued? Have you had a severe virus? ... ' and so on, '... then you may have Myalgic Encephalomyelitis ME.' Of course ME/CFS was little known and little publicised in 1985, and there was little or no research taking place in Australia then. I read on, all the symptoms mentioned related to me. I scribbled down the ME society's telephone number, which was listed, with the intention of contacting them immediately.

It turned out to be another landmark in my acceptance of my illness as it put me in touch with people in the same circumstances as myself, many of whom have become my friends. Anne and I, for instance, discovered we had the same doctor and the same chemical sensitivities so together we set about finding safe alternatives to the things which were sending us into relapse. We compared notes often and we have both, with the same treatment and approach, rehabilitated ourselves from being total invalids during long periods of severe relapse to leading fairly normal lives so long as we keep our environment clean and do not get too overtired.

The friendships I have made are very special. I have one particular friend who has been bedridden during all the time I have known her. She has been too sick to visit Dr Eric more than a couple of times because of her total lack of mobility and need for an ambulance to transport her. She has found small improvement on his remedies but alas has not been able to continue the treatment. I admire her strength of character as she lives alone and is mainly dependent on strangers to look after her. There must be many like sufferers in our community. It is often in these cases, where for any reason the family cannot rally around with practical support and loving care, that the ME/CFS sufferer faces an extremely difficult battle. After all, there is nothing in the world as wonderful as the love and care of one's family, where we truly belong, to assist the healing process.

Every crisis in our lives is a learning experience. I am sure it is a test to see how we will cope. It is interesting to see, in retrospect, that out of great suffering and sadness there will most often come, eventually, understanding, closeness and unexpected happiness. I think that if we adopt a positive attitude, and try not to feel sorry for ourselves for too long, we will find that there was a purpose in that crisis and learning experience which will be to our advantage in the future.

I have learnt so much about myself, about medicine, about the environment and the purpose of life since becoming ill, and I hope that I am in some small way passing on to you a frame of mind, hope, and some practical advice to help you to overcome your sicknesss.

I have also been strengthened by my belief that there is a Divine Being, God, directing our lives, and whilst always striving to do my best, have become fairly philosophical about life. A close friend handed me this prayer just at the time I was contemplating putting all I had learned about my illness onto paper. Together with Leonie's prompting, it was really the catalyst which enabled me to start writing.

God has created me to do Him some definite service. He has committed some work to me which He has not committed to another. I have my mission. I may never know it in this life, but I shall be told it in the next.

I am a link in a chain, a bond of connection between persons. He has not created me for naught. I shall try to do good, I shall do His work. I shall be an angel of peace, a preacher of truth in my own place while not intending it — if I do but keep His commandments.

Therefore, I will trust Him. Whatever, wherever I am. I can never be thrown away. If I am in sickness, my sickness may serve Him, in perplexity, my perplexity may serve Him. If I am in sorrow, my sorrow may serve Him. He does nothing in vain. He knows what He is about. He may take away my friends, make my spirits drop, hide my future from me; still He knows what He is about.

JOHN HENRY NEWMAN 1801–90

Relaxation, acupuncture and home remedies

Relaxation is a very necessary part of regaining health and staying healthy. Relaxation means different things to different people. Some like fishing, others like to paint or read, or even go for a stroll through the bush, maybe just sit on the beach and watch the waves breaking on the sand — each is relaxing in its own way. However, with our busy twentieth century lifestyles we often do not have the time necessary to provide for these periods of relaxation and so we keep the adrenalin pumping far more than nature intended.

I have not found it easy to relax. My central nervous system seems to have been affected in some way which makes relaxation more difficult to achieve, especially the 'feeling heavy' sensation. I fight against this particular technique because it feels as though I am going into relapse. However, I do take time out of each day to practice.

Relaxation can be practised in either a sitting or lying position. If you prefer sitting, sit with your back fairly straight, your head resting on the back of the chair or held straight, and your arms and hands resting on the arms of the chair, or with your hands in your lap (see fig. 1). If you prefer to lie down, lie on your back (a pillow under your knees will take the strain from your back) either on the floor or the bed, with your arms next to your body, palms upwards (see fig. 2). It is not essential to feel absolutely comfortable as, with practice of your preferred relaxation technique, the feeling of discomfort will spur you on to find deep relaxation wherein the discomfort will disappear. However, to begin with I would suggest that comfort be a consideration. Here are some techniques for you to try:

1   Lie down, or sit, in a comfortable postion, keeping warm, in a darkened room. Close your eyes and try to focus on a pinpoint of light. As it becomes clearer, try to see it as a *blue* light. Concentrate on this blue light and at the same time try to see it expanding and getting brighter. Try to keep it up for at least 10-20 minutes. Always return slowly from relaxation, bring your mind back to where you are in the room, move and stretch a little, then open your eyes.

2   Lie or sit in a comfortable position. Slowly picture each part of your body and, if you feel any tension, try to relax those muscles. Then, picture yourself transported to your favourite, most relaxing place. It might be sitting on the beach, watching a trout stream or in a rainforest. Just close your eyes and picture all of the surroundings and imagine the noises you would hear there. Relax your face, smile a little, and stay in your favourite place for as long as you can, at least for 10 minutes.

3   If you prefer, you can relax by concentrating on your breathing. Lie or sit in your favourite, most relaxed position. It is better if no parts of your body are touching and your muscles are not under tension. Take that frown off your face, let your jaw sag, take a deep breath

and sigh, close your eyes and concentrate solely on your breathing. If outside sounds disturb you, just start again. Continue for 10-20 minutes.

4   A similar technique can be practised by choosing a single word and repeating it over and over again, e.g. 'one, one, one . . .'

5   Remember also that you can achieve instant relaxation, even in the most tense situations, if you take a deep breath, sigh whilst breathing out and drop your shoulders, loosen up the face and jaw, even smile a little, and remember that getting uptight is not going to solve any situation, whatever it might be.

All this is easy to say, but it's not so easy to do. Practice does help, I can assure you of that. I would recommend you read Ian Gawler's book *You Can Conquer Cancer*, which gives complete instructions for 'healing meditations'. You might also find it helpful to attend a relaxation or stress management course run by your local community centre for health services.

The following are some tips for relieving pain and other common problems associated with ME/CFS. Some of them were given to me by Leonie who has an abundant store of practical ways to reduce pain, all of which can be practised at home.

Headache

Place an ice-cube on the very top of the head. To find the very top draw an imaginary line across the top of the head from ear to ear, then a line from the centre of the forehead to the back of the head — where the two lines cross is the centre of the head. Leave the ice cube there for about a minute (see figs. 3 & 4). Relief can be accelerated by placing the feet in fairly warm water at the same time. I have found this very helpful in relieving headaches when I occasionally get them.

A dose of homoeopathic Bryonia may also relieve a headache. Pressure or massage on the point in the V formed by the index finger and the thumb of your hand will also help — *always use pressure that is as strong as the pain.* (see figs. 5 & 6)

Soreness or stiffness of the back and neck

Fold a towel in half lengthwise. Roll it into a sausage. Lie on your back on the floor, put a pillow under the knees then place the rolled-up towel under your neck so that it supports your neck while your head is resting on the floor. Relax in that position (it should be very comfortable), for five minutes (see fig. 7). Gently roll to one side, then either sit or stand up straight (in front of a mirror preferably) and press the palm of your right hand firmly against the right side of your head just above the ear while holding your head straight (that is, upright and with the chin tucked in, not out) (see figs. 8, 9 & 10). Then do the same on the left side of the head and relax (see fig. 11); gently turn your head towards the right shoulder (see fig. 12), then towards the left shoulder (see fig. 13). You will be surprised how this can take the tension out of the neck and upper back.

Pain in lower back

Lie on your back on a mattress or padded mat, with pillows under your head and knees. Bring your knees up slowly, one at a time, towards your chest (see figs. 14 & 15). Place your hands on your knees then gently rock your knees backwards and forwards (see fig. 16). Do this in rhythm with your breathing, breathing *out* when your knees are moving toward your chest and breathing *in* while they're moving away from your chest. (Only do this about five times depending on your strength.)

If you're too weak for this exercise, roll into a foetal position on your side.

These exercises stretch the lower spine. Remember that the stomach muscles support the spine. When you are

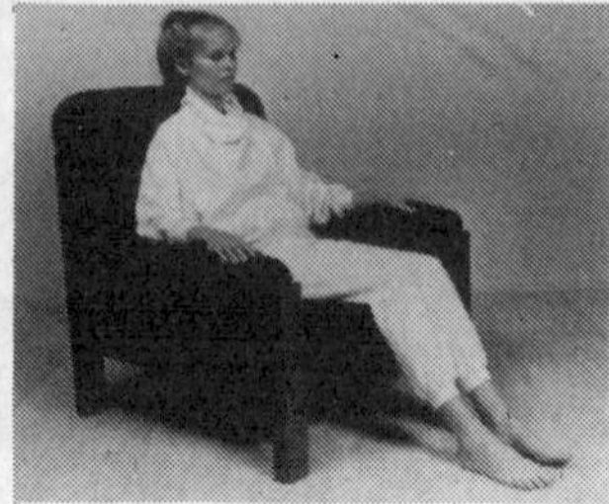

Figure 1 For relaxation

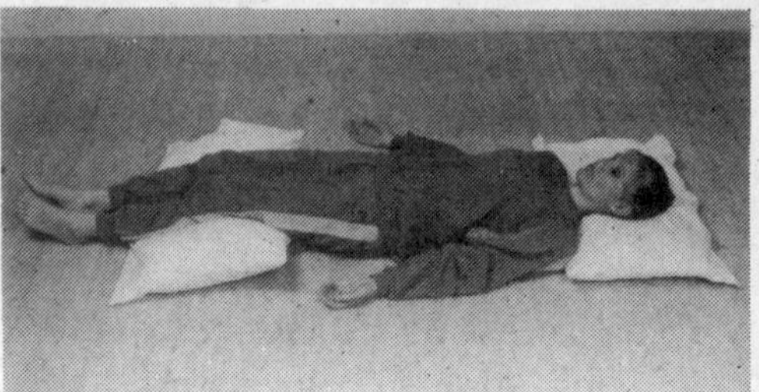

Figure 2 For relaxation

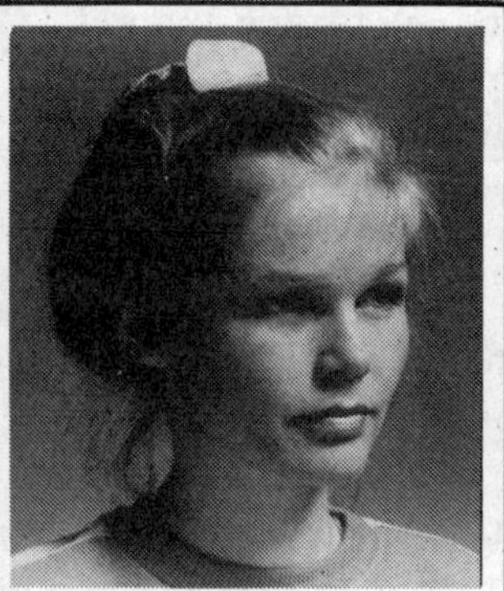

Figure 3 For headache

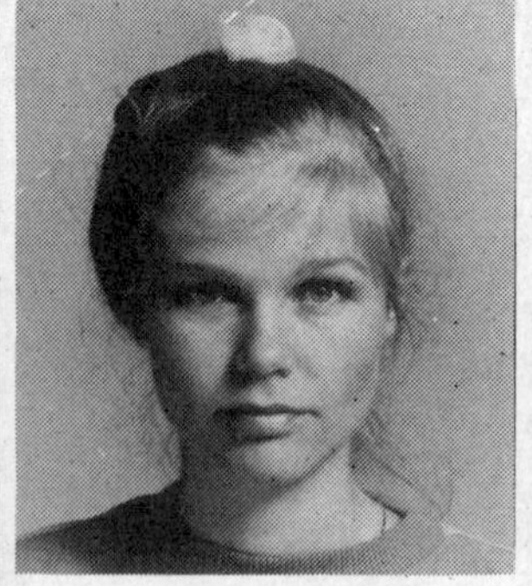

Figure 5 For headache

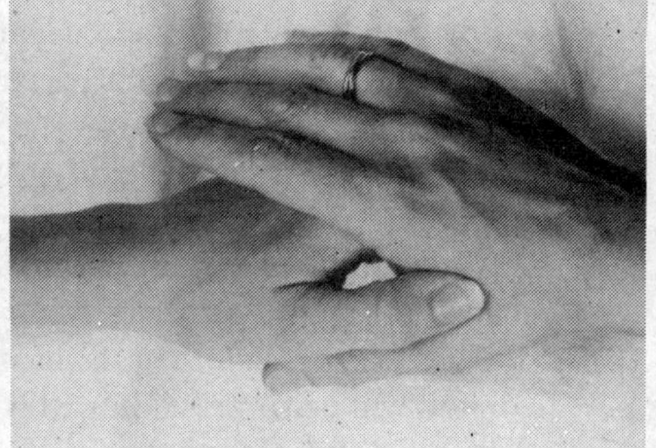

Figure 4 For headache

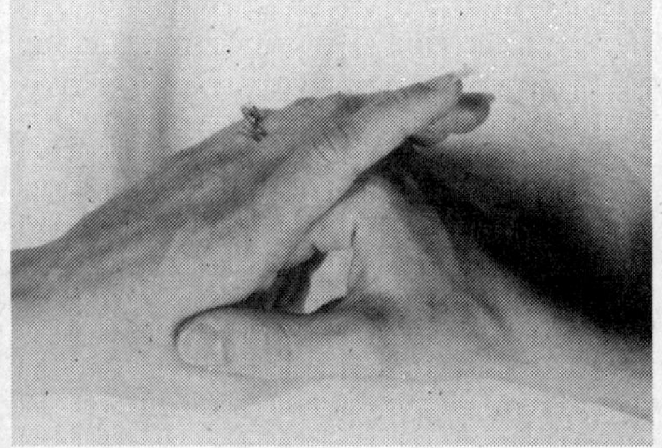

Figure 6 For headache

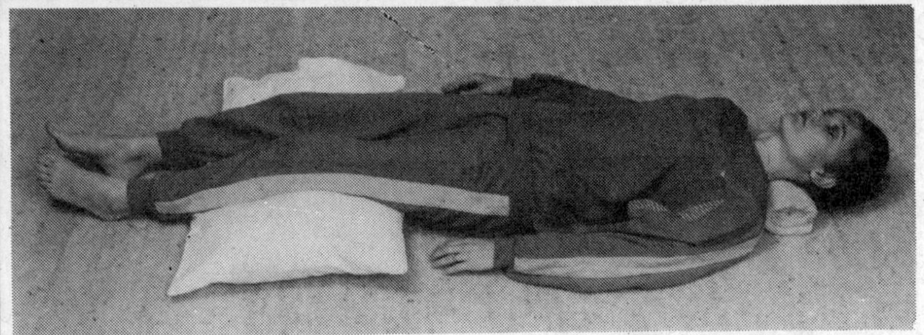

Figure 7 For back & neck pain

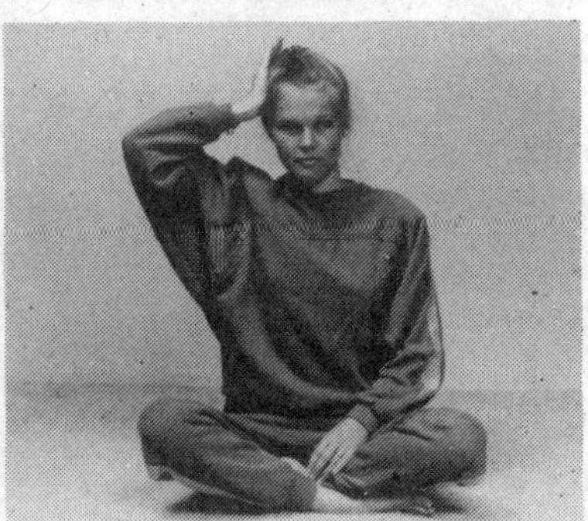

Figure 8 For back & neck pain

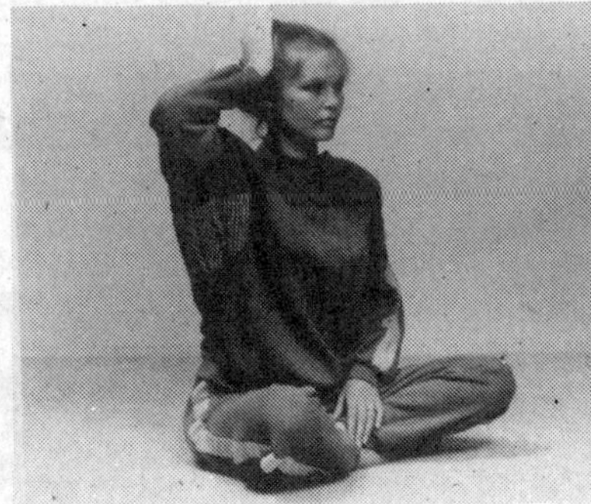

Figure 9 For back & neck pain
(side view)

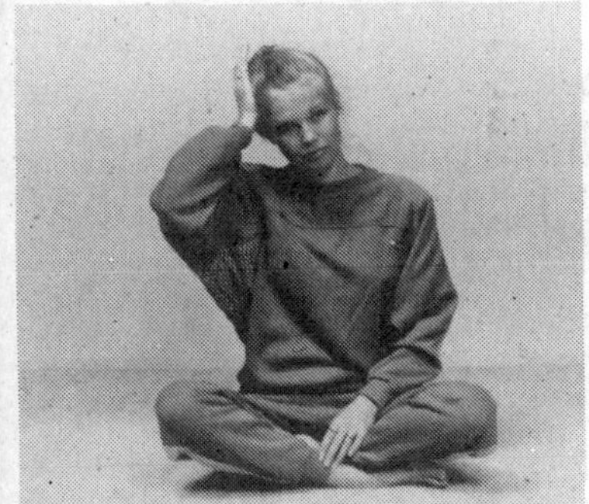

Figure 10 For back & neck pain
(incorrect position)

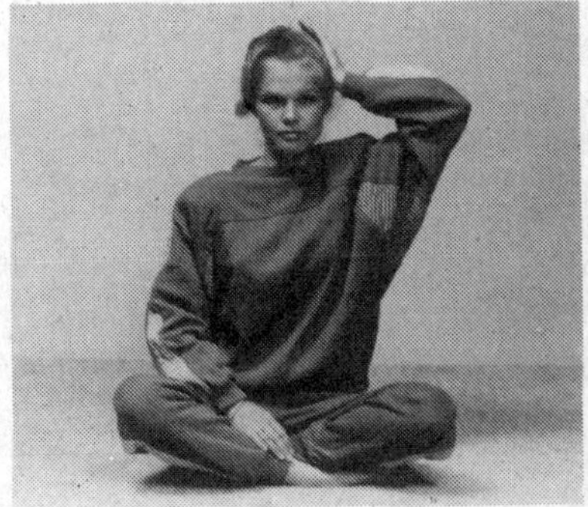

Figure 11 For back & neck pain

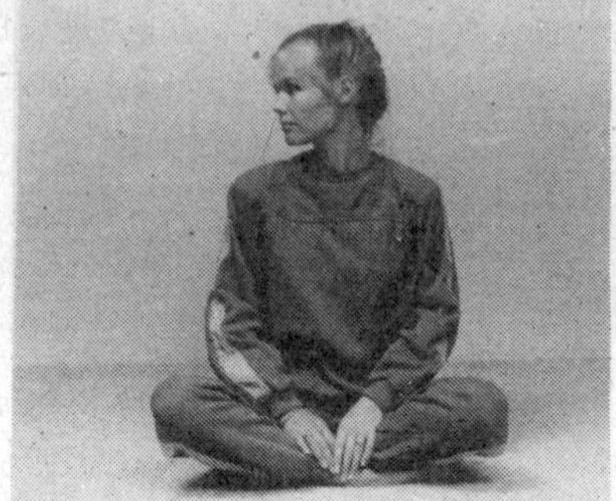

Figure 12 For back & neck pain

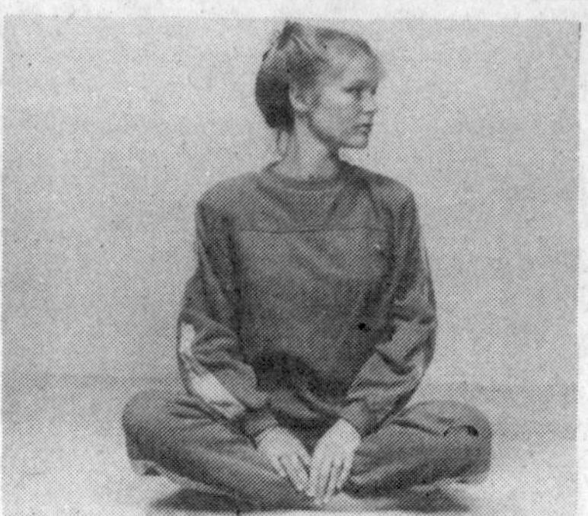

Figure 13 For back & neck pain

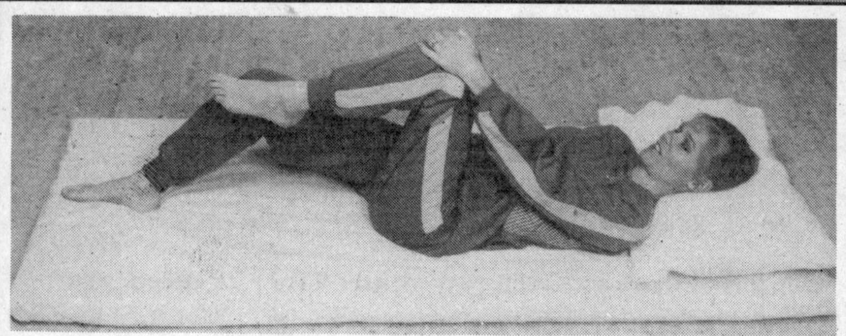

Figure 14 For lower back pain

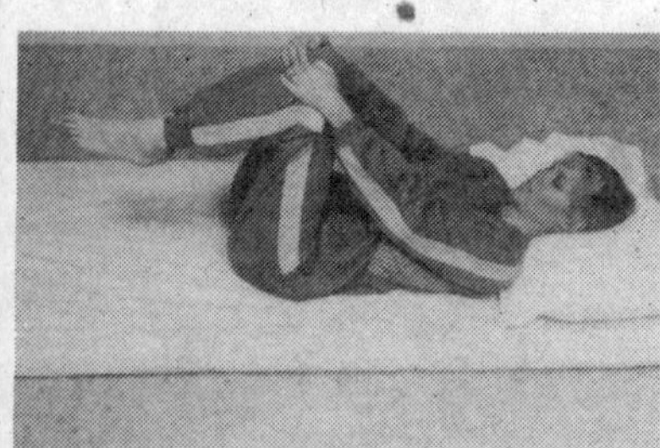

Figure 15 For lower back pain

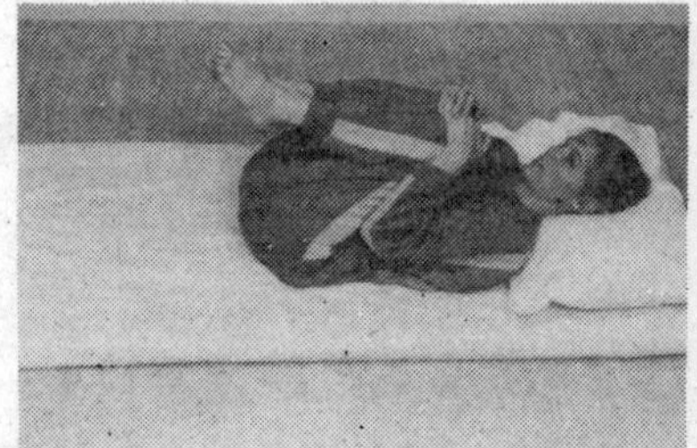

Figure 16 For lower back pain

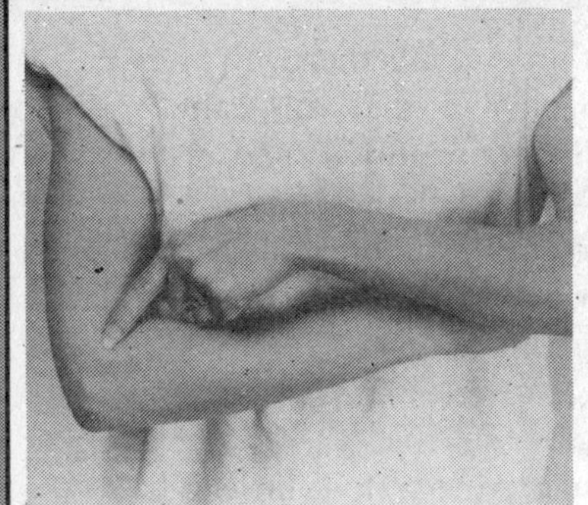
Figure 17 For leg cramps

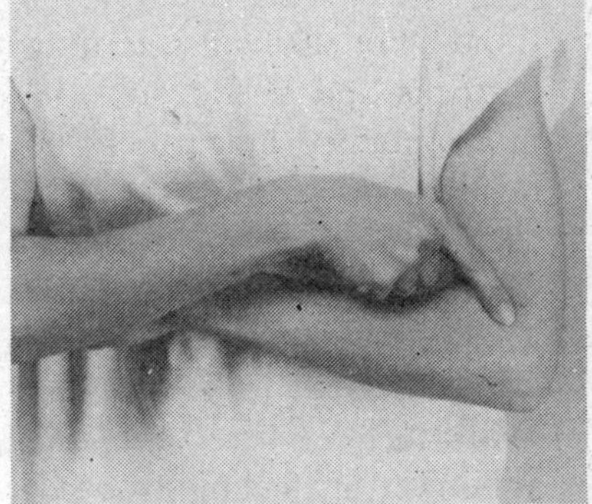
Figure 18 For leg cramps

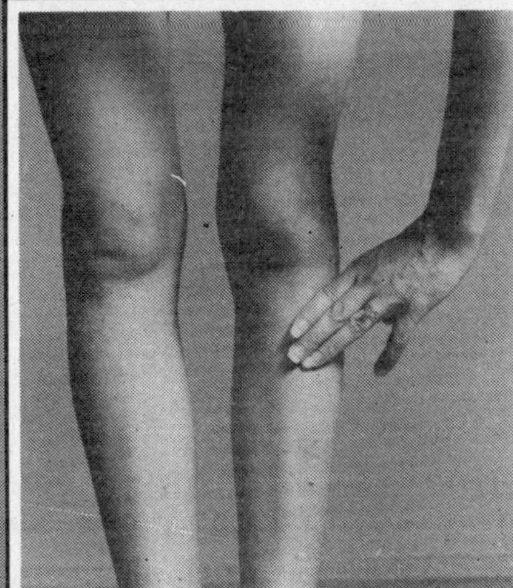
Figure 19 For upset stomach

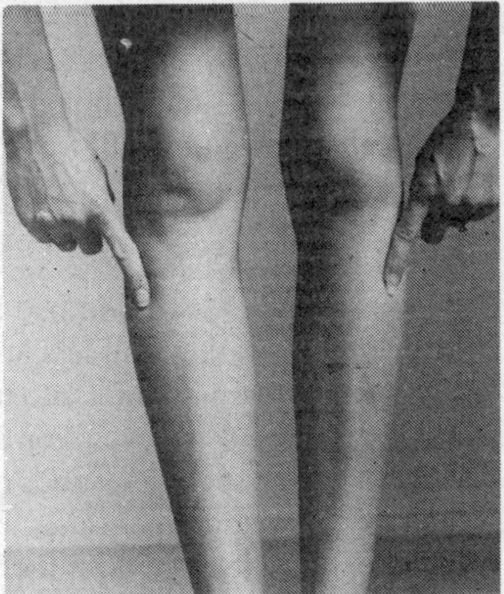
Figure 20 For upset stomach

standing or sitting, try to draw them in, together with your buttocks and pelvic area. It is obvious that this cannot be maintained indefinitely, but be conscientious and do it regularly rather than letting those stomach muscles slacken each day. Tense them when you are standing talking to someone, or any time you think of it. Strong stomach muscles will relieve a lot of back problems.

Walking

When you are feeling strong enough, try to go for a little walk each day — even if it is only 20 metres it is a start — being conscious of your deportment as you move. Swing your arms as though you were marching — this transfers energy from one side of the brain to the other. If you're unsure of your capabilities and worried about fatigue, marching on the spot at home will give you an indication of your stamina and ability to walk. Hasten slowly though, and do not attempt it if your legs feel fatigued as it will worsen your condition. Rather, do the exercises mentioned under 'Bedridden' below.

Bedridden

If you are forced to stay in bed for lengthy periods do gentle exercises by rotating your feet and wriggling your toes. Do the same with the arms, hands and fingers, so that the muscles do not become weak. Contraction and relaxation of each part of the body for about five seconds is of great assistance also. Roll over in bed a couple of times and loosen up your head and neck. (The rolled up towel technique already described will help here.) Depending on your level of fatigue, do some or all of these exercises a few times per day. It is important not to let the muscles waste too much. If a gentle, hand massage can be arranged it is very soothing and will help muscle tone. Avoid a vibrator/massager as this may cause fatigue.

Lymphatic drainage

This was mentioned in the first chapter and is most beneficial if you are bedridden. The lymphatics become congested when one is incapacitated and in order to get the fluids to drain from one gland to another, stroking massage is of great benefit. An osteopath will do this. Of course, walking will do the same thing, and that is why massage and bed-exercises are helpful when out of action.

Swimming

Those like myself who are lucky enough to possess a solar heated, non-chemical pool will find exercising in warm water wonderful. If you are not so lucky, take advantage of the summer months and swim gently in the ocean as much as possible — but stay away from pollution. I am sure this hydrotherapy has helped me enormously. Even just standing in the water will, as Dr Eric says 'earth you out'.

Baths or showers

Spending long periods in a steamy bathroom is not desirable. Chloroform is a low concentration by-product of chlorinated water and a bath is therefore preferable to a long shower. Make sure it is not too hot, otherwise this will cause fatigue. Leave the window open or use an exhaust fan to provide plenty of ventilation and make those ablutions as quickly as possible.

Cramps

For severe cramps in the legs, bend the elbow and find the spot at the end of the outside crease. It should feel sore and massaging it will relieve the cramp. For cramp in your left leg, massage your right arm (see fig. 17); for cramp in your right leg, massage your left arm (see fig. 18). (You are using acupressure!) A small amount of salt placed on the tongue is also helpful as is Dolomite powder — take one teaspoon on retiring.

Temperature

When running a temperature do not immediately think 'I must take aspirin and get it down'. To do this would be working against nature because a temperature is nature's way of fighting a virus or infection. Medication should be given only when it is dangerously high i.e. 38.5 or over for a child with no history of convulsions and 39.5 or over for an adult. Dr Eric informs me also that frail elderly people generally do not run a temperature.

The best way of treating a high temperature is to have a tepid sponge all over, or if you're well enough, a tepid shower or bath. This will make you much more comfortable. We have to learn to work *with* nature and so encourage and assist the healing processes.

Sore throat

For a sore throat which results from inhaling toxic fumes, a gargle with salt and purified water is very soothing. A few drops of calendula can be added. Spit out after gargling.

For a throat infection, gargle with pure lemon juice and swallow the juice. Do this three times daily *after* meals. Do not eat or drink anything for one hour after the gargle. Homoeopathic Strep/Staph 200, if available, is excellent as well.

Sore dry nose or catarrh

Add half a teaspoon of salt to one cup of warm, purified water. Pour it into the cupped palm of one hand and, holding the index finger of your other hand against the side of your nose to close the nostril, snuffle up the salty water into the open nostril; now throw your head back to allow the salty water to drain down the back of the throat. Repeat with the other nostril (don't drown yourself). Do this half a dozen times in each nostril and repeat every four hours if possible. (Swimming/diving in the ocean has a similar effect.) It is surprising how this will clear up catarrh and is very soothing for sore or dry nose problems.

When my nose and throat tell me that I have encountered nasty fumes, as soon as I return home I gargle and snuffle with salty water and drink a couple of glasses of purified water.

Upset Stomach

This is often due to either a germ, a digestive problem or thrush. A wonderful, soothing remedy is chamomile tea. Follow this up with Slippery Elm, either in powder or tablet form. It will soothe an inflamed stomach and is a marvellous remedy. Aloe Vera will do likewise. For diarrhoea, raw potato juice is most effective. (Chew pieces of raw potato and spit out the bulk.) Do not forget, like everything else the tummy or colon needs a rest to get better, so take only purified water with a little salt and sugar, and some chamomile tea, for a day or two (depending on the severity of the problem, especially if you have contracted a bug) before returning to food. Introduce foods slowly. Apples provide potassium and are excellent. Choose foods that are easily digestible such as potato, pasta, rice, squash, zucchini, pumpkin, pawpaw, marrow, chokos. Peppermint tea is good for gas or wind in the stomach and bowel. For an ongoing stomach problem, digestive enzymes may help. On your lower leg, three finger widths below the knee and between the tibia and the outside of your leg, there should be a sore spot (see figs. 19 & 20). Massage the soreness away on both legs and this should improve the tummy.

Fruit juices

These can cause digestive problems as they are fairly concentrated. Always dilute them, especially for children. Nature intended us to eat the whole fruit as this slows down the passage of the juices into the colon. A paediatrician from the Children's Hospital, Camperdown in Sydney blames apple juice and take-away chicken for the upsurge of bowel problems in children.

Acupuncture

A skilled acupuncturist can be very soothing to the ME/CFS sufferer. Checking the pulses and balancing the energies of the body can bring great relief. It is not absolutely necessary to have the needles as the laser (low frequency divergent beam) is also very effective. I have visited Leonie with a very distressed digestive system, feeling very uptight, and left her feeling calm and out of pain. She precedes her treatments with a hand massage which is absolutely wonderful.

Foot massage

This can be very beneficial, both by way of soothing the feet and stimulating various organs of the body. Massage the foot gently all over, using olive oil, then concentrate your efforts on the sole of the foot. Work gently until you discover a 'sore spot'. Work on that spot until the soreness has disappeared. You may find extremely tender spots, so start gently and increase the pressure of the massage gradually. This is very beneficial when bedridden. It is better for someone other than the patient to perform this massage.

Sleeplessness

This seems to be a dreadful problem for many ME/CFS sufferers, particularly when in severe relapse. I cannot offer a real solution except putting your feet into hot water, having a warm drink of milk and relaxing before bedtime. Homoeopathic Gelsemium was helpful for me and so was tuning into the radio or reading. I tried Valerian and L-Tryptophan but they did not seem to work. I've suffered with this problem for many years but I found that as soon as I really started to regain my health I began sleeping again.

Panic attacks and Agoraphobia

Panic attacks can strike at any time. Worrying about whether you will get a panic attack can also trigger one off. If you happen to be struck with a panic attack, hold your breath for five seconds (count slowly to five) and then concentrate on taking even breaths but not more than ten or twelve per minute. This will help you to relax. (This programme is taught at the Agoraphobia Clinic St Vincents Hospital, Sydney).

Recent research shows that sufferers of this problem have a deficiency of a chemical in the brain, and according to a professor I heard being interviewed on the radio, once that chemical is replaced by medication, and control of the attacks is taught by relaxation, there is a great hope of improvement. In other words, this is a physiological disorder, not necessarily a mental one.

Check up with Gynaecologist

If you are chemically sensitive, be careful about any lubricants or sterilising agents used on instruments which come in contact with the mucous membranes. I broke out in a dreadful rash after my last examination. The gynaecologist was mystified as he had never seen anything like it and pathology tests revealed nothing. Dr Eric thought it may have been an allergic reaction to the sterilising solution on the instruments. It is wise to take your own natural live culture yogurt to use as a lubricant and to make sure that the instruments are thoroughly rinsed before insertion.

Antibiotics

Antibiotics should be avoided unless we are faced with a very serious illness. They seem to have a particularly adverse effect on ME/CFS sufferers. As well as destroying the 'unhealthy' bacteria, antibiotics destroy 'healthy' bacteria such as lactobacillus, acidophilus and bulgaricus, which often results in an outbreak of thrush/candida because the bowel flora has been altered. It is essential, when taking antibiotics, to replace those 'healthy' bacteria. This can be done by eating lots of *live culture* yogurt. There are many brands of living culture yogurt available at health food stores. Acidophilus tablets are also an excellent source of these healthy bacteria and will help minimise the side effects of the antibiotics.

Medications

Note: This advice does not apply to homoeopathic remedies.

Avoid taking any tablets or medicines, including vitamin tablets, when lying down. Always sit up and allow time for them to pass down the oesophagus into the stomach. Unless otherwise stipulated, tablets and medications should be taken with food so as to minimise their effects on the stomach lining.

My husband recently underwent extensive leg surgery which required pretty strong pain-killers for some weeks afterwards. He would not take any notice of me when I suggested the above. However, he learnt the hard way as he experienced pain and burning in the throat and oesophagus plus indigestion problems. In the end he resorted to suppositories to ease the pain and it took some months for those digestive disturbances to clear up.

Worms

Soak ½ cup dried pumpkin seeds in lemon juice and garlic (4 cloves) overnight. Eat over a period of 3 days. (Use 6–8 seeds for children.) There are also some homoeopathic remedies for worms including Cina, Santoninum and Spigelia.

Head Lice

Boil two tablespoons of 'Quassia chips' with one cup of water. To wash your hair with this solution, rub it into hair and scalp, leave it on hair and cover with shower cap for half an hour; rinse; shampoo hair in usual way. 'Quassia chips' can be purchased from some chemists and health food stores. Castor oil and sassafras oil left on the hair overnight will also do the trick. A Tea Tree Oil massage will also help.

Combing with a fine comb and keeping the hair clean will certainly help the situation. Head lice may be a nuisance but will not cause a serious health problem and it seems to me that some preparations sold for the treatment of head lice are much more harmful than the lice themselves.

Arthritis

A copper bracelet is now proven to be beneficial. Two doctors in Newcastle set out to disprove this 'old wives tale' only to find that it works scientifically. A copper ointment called 'Alcusal' (available from chemists) has the same effect, but because it is concentrated and in an ointment base, it does cause a reaction on the skin of some people. Use only an amount equivalent to the size of your little fingernail.

Homoeopathic Arnica and Arnica ointments are very helpful with arthritis.

Electromagnetic clips are also helpful. (See Directory page 224).

Reactions

If you wish to know whether you will react unfavourably to something, put a small amount on the inside of your wrist. Leave it on for several hours, or overnight, and if there is no redness, burning or reaction of any kind it is pretty safe in general.

Burns

As soon as you receive a severe burn, immerse it in icy cold water (but do not put ice directly on the burn). When the skin has cooled sufficiently, apply Aloe Vera. If you have a plant growing, cut off a piece of the fleshy leaf, peel apart and extract the colourless glue-like substance from between the flesh. Cover the area with this. Homoepathic Cantharis and Arnica given at this time will relieve pain and blistering.

'Burn Cream' from Martin and Pleasance is very good as an alternative. (See Ointments page 160.)

Fingernails

If infections around the fingernails are a problem, the following is a recipe my mother used when I was a child. It is extremely effective and I have recently used it for this purpose. Mix together one tablespoon of flour, one teaspoon of honey and enough white of an egg to make a paste. Apply the paste generously using lint and bandage the finger. Replace the paste twice daily. Your finger should begin to heal within a couple of days.

Splinters and thorns

Honey can be used to draw out splinters or thorns, especially if they are causing infection. Honey will draw out infection and reduce inflammation. It will also draw out blackheads.

Blue bottle and jelly fish stings

Always keep a small bottle of vinegar handy when swimming in the ocean or lake etc. as this will negate the toxins in such stings. Do not rub sand onto the sting or apply methylated spirit as this will maximise the effects of the poison. If stung in the mouth, tongue, neck etc. and swelling occurs, ice (a paddle pop will suffice) will help to slow the swelling and possible asphyxiation until medical attention can be found.

Masks

Although it may seem embarrassing I find my mask invaluable when confronted with an unexpected 'situation'. When I apologised and donned it in a waiting room, the cigarette smokers all put their cigarettes out. Having to shop in newly painted premises is much less hazardous when wearing a mask. On such occasions I have received a few 'smart alec' remarks which I have countered immediately and sent the culprit scurrying. Remember, we are not second class citizens because we have allergies! As we never know when we may encounter pesticide or herbicide sprays or other toxic fumes it is a good idea to keep masks in a handy place, namely, in the pocket or handbag. To obtain masks see Charcoal Masks page 159.

There are many more helpful hints in 'How to Minimise Exposure to Toxic Chemicals', page 142-185, as well as alternative products.

Thrush or Candida

Candida seems to be a problem with modern living. It is triggered off in many cases by antibiotics and other drugs which deplete the body of healthy bacteria.

Candida (Thrush) attacks the mucous membranes and can make itself obvious in the mouth or genital area. However, quite often it attacks the colon or bowel and you can be unaware of its presence except that digestive and bowel problems may be evident.

The ME seminar held by the Australian Medical Faculty of Homoeopathy in 1987 included intense discussion on candida and its suspected implication in the ME/CFS syndrome. Dr John, a colleague of Dr Eric's, who spoke on the relationship between candida and ME, stated that his investigations had found that cell wall deficient bacteria/organisms called L-forms were present in significant numbers in the blood of people who were immune compromised. In his talk he explained that when the bowel flora is altered, the bacteria which normally keep the candida under control, are insufficient to do the job and the candida (which is a yeast) grows out of control and alters the lining of the bowel. By eating foods which feed the candida, such as sugar, yeast and moulds, the problem is further aggravated. Thus, the lining of the colon/bowel, which protects us from many proteins and bacteria, becomes leaky and macro-molecules (food particles and food proteins), including candida organisms, sneak through into the bloodstream resulting in a diagnosis of 'Systemic Candida'. Dr John further pointed out that it is not just the candida but also the food particles and food proteins which are being allowed to sneak into the blood stream that are causing further problems.

If you suspect thrush to be a problem, first establish whether it is systemic or not. This can be achieved by having a blood test (Darkfield Live Blood Analysis), which your medical practitioner should organise. If the result indicates systemic candida, your doctor will prescribe Nystatin to clear candida from within the colon and/or Ketoconazole to remove it from the blood. Intravenous Vitamin C has been used successfully in some people. If you have thrush and it is not systemic (not in the bloodstream) then adopting the following practices should eventually clear it up:

- Avoid yeast (bread, cakes, pastries, buns).
- Avoid moulds (mushrooms, cheese, dried fruits, melons).
- Avoid sugar.
- Take acidophilus tablets as prescribed and/or eat lots of natural (live culture) yogurt.
- A few doses of homoeopathic candida works in many cases but not all.
- Take one teaspoon of olive oil three times per day before meals. Olive oil is a wonderful food, does not contain cholesterol and is marvellous for all types of fungus infections.
- Take one or two teaspoons of cod liver oil each day, first thing in the morning or last thing at night. If you cannot stomach that, buy the cod liver oil gelatin capsules available at health food stores. Remember, cod liver oil is rich in Vitamin A which helps keep the mucous membranes healthy.

Some practitioners recommend two drops of Tea Tree oil (this could be added to the olive oil) by mouth three times per day (but only two drops as it is toxic in excessive doses). Tea Tree oil is great for fungus infections.

If the genital area (female) is the problem, then live culture natural yogurt used internally will clear it up. Buy a few pieces of 'natural sea sponge' from the chemist, cut it to the approximate size of a tampon to suit you, wash the sponge well with warm water and pure soap, rinse well — you can add two drops of Tea Tree oil to the rinsing water — squeeze well, dip into natural yogurt (not flavoured) and insert into vagina just before going to bed. The bacteria in live culture yogurt are the same as those occurring naturally in your body. (Incidentally, I am at the menopause stage and I find that yogurt applied to the surrounding mucous areas of the vagina each day keeps it moist and healthy.)

Wearing loose-fitting undergarments made from cotton which breathes is also very important as fungus infections are encouraged in warm, moist conditions. Although they might be considered sexy by some, tight-fitting briefs and jeans should be avoided.

A typical diet for myself was as follows. Please take it only as a guide as each diet has to be individually tailored to your own specific food allergies and these can only be worked out by yourself (an elimination diet can be found in Dr Mackarness's *Chemical Victims*). I followed this programme for about six to twelve months and actually gained weight which surprised me as I was eating virtually no bread.

No dairy products, wheat, yeast (bread), onions, garlic, shallots, potatoes, pumpkin, beetroot, tomatoes, nuts, dried fruits, sugar, honey (no fruit for first month).

BREAKFAST   Demeter rolled oats (and stewed
                             apples after first month)

or

Polenta and fruit

or

Fresh fruit

Chamomile tea or Verbena tea

MORNING TEA — Piece of fruit and/or Kavli biscuits

LUNCH — Salad vegetables with egg or small quantity cold meat

or

Rice and salad

or

Salad and fruit with Kavli biscuits

AFTERNOON TEA — Dandelion coffee (with soy milk) and Rice crackers

DINNER — Vegetable soup

Small quantity meat, fish or chicken (free range), rice and green vegetables in season, steamed.

Stewed or fresh fruit

or

Consomme

Small quantity of meat, fish or chicken with salad or Chinese-style vegetables, stir fried

Baked apples with home made custard (soy milk) or fresh fruit salad

PLENTY OF PURIFIED WATER BETWEEN MEALS

Re-Introduce foods over 6–9 months.

The above is only a very basic example from the range of meals I prepare — I like cooking. Provided I do not eat packaged foods, preservatives and food additives but eat only organically grown grains, meat, fruit and vegetables, I do not seem to have severe food allergies. It's best not to eat too much of any one kind of vegetable or fruit. For example too many orange-coloured fruit and vegetables consumed in one day or on successive days can cause a problem because of an excess of beta-carotene. Try to rotate foods as much as possible.

It is not a good idea to totally and permanently eliminate culprit foods from the diet as this eventually may make a person more allergic, thus restricting their chemical tolerances even further. Therefore, every now and again have a little of the food which you really crave, always remembering that if swelling of the face or throat or other serious food reactions do occur, then absolute abstinence may be essential.

Rotation of food is the key to success.

It is interesting to note that whereas I really loved bread and ate it with almost every meal, I can now take it or leave it and I actually find that the taste is nowhere near as delicious as it used to be. That is not necessarily because of the quality of the bread (as I am able to purchase bread without additives) but because my taste buds seem to have changed.

I hope the above programme will work as well for you as it did for me. Be patient, however — it does take time.

How to minimise exposure to toxic chemicals

There is no doubt that avoiding exposure to toxic chemicals must be advantageous to everyone's health, so why not try it? It is so easy. If anyone had told me ten years ago that I could live without cleaning powders, tile cleaners, bleach and napthalene I would never have believed them, but I am living without them and I don't miss them one bit. My house and bathrooms are squeaky clean. I work on the theory that if toxic chemicals seem to be contributing to my illness, I should eliminate them as much as possible, as many of them are cumulative and every little exposure and absorption builds up. Also, by changing my lifestyle in this way I am not adding as much to the pollution problem by putting toxic chemicals into the sewers and drains, nor the land and air.

On the following pages I will try to suggest ways you can clean up your environment and alternative products to use and wear. I hope they will be of use to you. Remember, also, that if you have small children, their immune systems are very fragile, taking several years to develop. Exposure to and absorption of toxins may have serious consequences for them in the future. I only wish I had known these facts 30 years ago. My children would be a lot healthier.

A word of warning. — I have found the following advice and the products mentioned to be safe or tolerable, however each of us is different and there is no guarantee you will tolerate all of them. Some of the products are available Australia-wide, others are localised.

A *word of caution.* — Do not think that *all* the products sold at health food stores are petrochemical and formaldehyde-free, nor are they organically grown. In fact some of the shampoos, deodorants, cosmetics, etc. sold in health food stores do contain those chemicals. I can only recommend the ones I have investigated and believe to be safe. There are new products coming out every day, so in a short space of time there will be many new products not available to me at the time of writing. My purpose is to encourage you to read the labels and carry out your own investigations, and to let you know that non-toxic products are available if you take the trouble to find them. The more we demand them, the more they will be produced. Some of the chemists are now stocking herbal remedies and alternative medicines.

To protect yourself in general, adopt the following practices:
- Avoid any smell which makes you agitated, vague or dizzy, gives you sore or watery eyes, makes your nose/throat sore, affects your breathing, makes you feel nauseated, causes sudden weakness, headache or blurred vision, or any smell which *you dislike intensely.*
- Avoid any product which burns or irritates your skin, causes rashes or blotching.
- Avoid any foods which give you indigestion, heartburn, diarrhoea, stomach-ache, hives or rashes, bloating, palpitations, headache, asthma, hyperactivity, and any which you love, crave or hate.
- Avoid drugs and patent medicines generally, if possible. As stated previously many contain phenol and/or formaldehyde as well as volatile aromatic and chlorinated solvents and a few contain pesticides. Always check the

chemical composition of the medication with the chemist or drug company and ask them about possible side effects.

In summary, many of the following products contain either pesticides, insecticides, petrochemicals, formaldehyde, volatile aromatic or chlorinated solvents, glycol ethers or other toxic chemicals:

Drugs and patent medicines, rubber products, strong smelling glues and solvents, particle board, mothballs, napthalene, pest strips and sprays, self-carboning paper, pool chlorine, bleach, detergents, disinfectants containing phenol, mouthwashes, white out (water-based just tolerable), felt marking pens, new glossy magazines and newspapers, water proofing, deodorisers, bleached and perfumed toilet paper, disposable nappies, tampons, deodorised sanitary pads, petrol, diesel, kerosene, benzene, phenol, creosote, tar, wood stains, paints generally, cigarette smoke, gas fumes (especially unflued gas heaters), new carpet, garden sprays and weed treatments, (except natural and herbal), pressure pack sprays, cleaning fluids, synthetic fabrics, plastics, vinyl, air-conditioners, car polishes, new leather, inorganic fertilisers (some organic fertilisers contain chemical stabilisers), rat poisons, baby oil, paraffin, vaseline, petroleum jelly, tissues, cosmetics and toiletries, dry cleaning fluids, ammonia, mineral turps, fumigants.

'How can I live?' you ask. 'Very simply and easily,' I answer. It is just a matter of changing old habits and introducing new ones. Isn't it worth it to stay well?

You will be making your own personal contribution to cleaning up pollution. After all, our grandmothers or great-grandmothers used only the most basic of cleaning materials — pure soap, bi-carb and vinegar — plus elbow grease. I can remember scrubbing the floor with soap and water when I was a child — it is very good exercise and certainly does a thorough job! We also had a 'soap shaker' where we placed pieces of left over soap and this was used to wash the dishes. How things have changed! Therefore, if many of the products on the following pages are too expensive keep this in mind.

Alternative products, advice and treatments

Clothing and footwear

Avoid synthetic fabrics as much as possible. Purchase only cotton, linen, wool or silk, and remember that most of these have now been treated with formaldehyde to make the material stiff, crease-resistant, shrink-proof, moth-proof etc. and you should wash them before you wear them.

Try to buy only leather or canvas shoes; because of the treatment of leather you may find that some shoes have an offensive smell. Try to air them outside for a few days as the sun helps to 'blow out' the fumes. Avoid rubber and plastic shoes where possible, as they often create severe tinea and other fungal or dermatitis problems due to the sweating. It is good to go barefooted where practical and safe as this exercises the foot properly.

In and around the house

Painting, decorating and furnishing

Try to choose only natural fabrics such as wool, cotton, linen and silk. New carpets can be a real problem, particularly the berber type carpets, which seem to take months to 'blow out' so be careful when choosing carpet. Do not choose a rubber underlay. Have it put down during the summer months when you can open the house and air it constantly. When we built our little cottage on the mid-north coast we encountered many problems with fumes from the paints, stains, varnishes and carpet. At that stage I had only just realised my sensitivities and had not researched the safer products.

A tiled floor is the safest, cleanest and easiest to maintain. However, if you must have a carpet, follow the above suggestions.

Linoleum is making a comeback. Lino is made from natural products, cork, linseed oil and jute. Unlike vinyl flooring it will break down in the environment and will not cause pollution. In Europe it is an offence to dump PVC flooring — it has to be taken to a registered incinerator and burnt at extremely high temperature. This is to avoid toxins from the PVC flooring leaching into the water supplies in the years to come.

Ask at leading specialist floor covering stores for information on linoleum. Manufactured by DLW Flooring Systems (see Directory page 208).

Avoid laminated timber and chipboard as these can contain formaldehyde and/or volatile solvents in the glue and take ages to 'blow out'.

If wallpapering, sugar soap is odourless for cleaning down walls. Apply 'size' to the walls and put up a pre-pasted wallpaper, but don't use vinyl. Check with the manufacturer to see if the wallpaper paste has been treated with an anti-fungal preparation. You should not have to move out for this exercise. Choose wisely and be cautious.

Anti-mould preparations are not recommended, instead wash the area with bi-carb, sugar soap or borax. Be careful to wear gloves with the latter two. Avoid chlorine bleach, try a little vinegar or peroxide instead.

Painting can be a real problem. However, there is a range of non-toxic paints, varnishes, lacquers, stains and polishes made from raw materials of plants and trees, natural bonding agents, resins and waxes on the market. They are a little more costly than other ranges, but are well worth it. They are available from Bio-Products Australia Pty Ltd or their distributors (see Directory for addresses page 208-209).

If you are wise you will vacate the house completely when having extensive painting undertaken. Choose the least toxic paint and allow time for the fumes to 'blow out' before you return. Oil paints will take ages to 'blow out', and should be avoided.

Except for Bio-Products, most paints are toxic to some degree. You will find it helpful, if in doubt, to purchase a small can of the paint you have selected and paint a piece of board with that paint. Use a mask and do it outside. Bring the board inside, into a small room, (bathroom or laundry) and leave it there for a few hours with the door closed. Upon re-entering the room, observe your body's reactions. Is the smell intolerable? Does it affect your eyes, nose or throat? Does it make your chest tight, breathing tight, head ache or make you feel vague, dizzy, agitated or unable to concentrate? If the smell is intolerable, persevere no more. However, if you think it is tolerable, stay in the room for some time to see if you have any of the other reactions.

If you do decide to use the paint, you should still take precautions: avoid the fumes as much as possible, and never sleep in a room that has been freshly painted. Allow at least a week (or two weeks if possible) for water-based paints, and much longer for oil paints. You will have to make the judgement for yourself as the many brands of paints on the market take varying amounts of time to 'blow out'. You will soon know whether the fumes are affecting you because you will feel very tired the next day, especially if it happens to be your bedroom. It is important to protect babies and young children from paint fumes, so if you cannot afford to move out, paint one room at a time, making sure you keep the internal doors closed, and do not occupy the room until the fumes have dissipated. It is always better to be overcautious than to be sorry later. If you can afford them, Bio-Products paints and stains are obviously the answer. Even so, some natural oils and terpenes are not tolerated if you have petrochemical sensitivities so proceed with caution and let your body be your guide.

According to some household paint manufacturers, acrylic

paints cannot be manufactured without glycol ethers. However, the ACTU on behalf of the Seamans Union in Victoria, took this matter up with the manufacturers of paints used on ships because of the serious health problems caused by glycol ethers, particularly in confined spaces. The paints now contain methyl ethyl ketone instead. Masks and protective clothing are worn. (*Health and Safety at Work*, J. Matthews, 1985).

Further excellent ranges of safe indoor and outdoor paints, Aglaia and Livos, are being imported from Germany by Ecological Building and Living of Blackheath, NSW (Address in Directory). A telephone inquiry will give the distributors in each State. These paints are used in schools and hospitals in Germany for safety reasons.

Whether or not you have ME/CFS I would advise wearing a mask if doing any painting or decorating where fumes are apparent. Industrial carbon filter masks are available from the ME Society of NSW (see page 159).

Bedroom

Keeping your bedroom free from toxic chemicals is all important as so much is absorbed while we sleep.

Be careful when buying a new mattress as some are treated with moth-proofing and conditioning chemicals — choose one which does not smell. Mattress casings are available from Allersearch as well as cotton pillows, blankets and quilts (see Directory) but they are expensive. Alternatively, put two large blankets over the mattress, tucking them in well, and then two cotton sheets — this should do the trick. Put mattresses out in the sun to air as much as possible.

Do not buy foam rubber articles of any kind for your bedroom, and keep all furnishings in natural materials. Tontine pillows are odourless but I will settle for a feather-down pillow any day. Use cotton or woollen blankets (wash before using). A lambswool underblanket is truly recommended for comfort, however you will probably have to wash it first. I did. A feather-down continental quilt is another luxury if you can tolerate the feathers. Always air bedding and bedclothes frequently in the sun.

Don't bring dry cleaning into the bedroom. Always hang it outside to allow fumes to blow out before putting it away.

Kitchen, bathroom and laundry

I can highly recommend Herbon products manufactured by Herbonics Australia (address in Directory page 209). While they are a little expensive, they do not contain formaldehyde, terpenes, phenols, chlorine, organic mercurials, balsams, aluminium complexes, chloroflurocarbons, nor lanoline or beeswax. They have been produced in conjunction with the Allergy Association and are designed to be non-allergenic and non-pollutant. They are not perfumed.

Caring products are similar to Herbon except that the range is not as extensive and most are slightly perfumed with either natural lemon, eucalyptus or lavender oil. They are available from most Woolworths/Safeways Stores in the 'health bar' section. They are manufactured by Caring Products of Victoria (address in Directory).

Both Herbon and Caring Laundry Powder and Herbon Dishwasher Powder contain a small quantity (6%) phosphate and their products are mostly packaged in plastic. Each company has promised to look at the possibility of using a system of refilling containers at the retail stores (as does The Body Shop) so as to cut down the plastic pollution problems. Hopefully the retailers will co-operate.

Brot Bodyline of New South Wales (address in Directory) manufacture from natural oils and rainwater lye, pure Soap, Shampoo Bar and Laundry Powder (needs washing soda added to wash) which are gentle, non-perfumed, non-allergenic and the packaging is environmentally-friendly. Available at health food stores. (New product so ask.)

Sunlight Velvet Soap and (laundry) Soap Powder, manufactured by Lever & Kitchen do not contain either petrochemicals, formaldehyde or phosphate. They are made from beef fat (tallow) and perfumed slightly with citronella. The laundry powder does contain a chemical 'optical brightener'; however, since meeting with the Managing Director and General Development Manager I have been told there is a 'high possibility' that the brightener will be removed from the product. Both products have environmentally-safe packaging. Lever and Kitchen are looking at their other products with regard to phosphate content, perfumes and environmentally safe packaging.

Dishwashing
I can recommend Herbon and Caring Dishwashing Liquids, Nutri-Clean O.L.C., from Nutri-metics, Herbon Botanical soap and Sunlight/Velvet laundry soap.

Dishwasher
Herbon Dishwashing Machine Powder. (Although this dishwashing powder is expensive to purchase it contains no chlorine and lasts me for five months.)

General
For general cleaning of sink, benches, baths, basins, shower recess etc., sprinkle bi-carb as you would a powdered cleaner. Rub some laundry soap (Sunlight/Velvet) on a moistened sponge and use with the bi-carb; rinse thoroughly. This will clean almost anything and will not scratch. The sink may need an extra amount of bi-carb and a scrub with a brush. It's an excellent method for the shower recess and does not seem to encourage mould, which should be treated with vinegar. Herbon also make a multi-purpose cleaner. Use Herbon detergent for washing floors or scrub them with laundry soap and water.

Toilet
Clean as recommended above. Vinegar is also recommended. Disinfect with a couple of drops of Tea Tree oil or

eucalyptus (if you can tolerate it). Avoid toilet fresheners and disinfectants as many contain chemicals which may upset you and add to pollution.

Laundry powders and liquids
I recommend Herbon Soap Powder, Bionomics Aware and Caring Laundry Powder (eucalyptus), Herbon and Caring Laundry Liquid, Sunlight/Velvet Laundry Powder. Be sure not to inhale any laundry powders when putting them in the washing machine. Either wear a mask or hold your breath. *Save suds*, to re-use in the next load as much as possible.

Use soap powder sparingly. Soak clothes overnight in cold water with soap powder to remove stains. A little bi-carb and soap rubbed on stains is efficient or Herbon Pre-Wash Stain Remover. For very stained whites; grease and inbuilt stains can be removed by boiling the clothes in a pot on the stove with a little soap powder. Place the clothes and powder in cold water, bring them to boil and boil for half an hour. Peroxide can be used to bleach stubborn stains.

Woollens: Handwash woollen garments in either Herbon Laundry or Dishwashing Liquid or Brot Bodyline soap. Add some lavender oil or eucalyptus oil to the last rinse. This will help to keep the moths at bay. Store woollens in a bag with either dried lavender or sage. Alternatively, a few drops of lavender oil on a piece of cotton wool tucked in with the woollens will do.

Cleaning
Refrigerator
You won't beat bi-carb for this chore. Moisten sponge, dip into bi-carb and rub onto all surfaces. It will help to deodorise as well as clean. Rinse thoroughly and add a little vanilla (pure essence) to the rinse if desired.

Oven cleaning
Mix bi-carb with a little water until it forms a paste equivalent to light starch. Apply with sponge to all surfaces of inside of

oven. Warm oven. The grease will wipe off. If oven is very dirty, put quite a thick paste of bi-carb onto it and leave for a few hours after warming. A wooden scraper will not scratch when removing thick patches of grease. When clean, re-coat oven with a very light paste of bi-carb. This will protect it from grease when cooking and make the job so much easier next time. The oven should not need much more than a wipe-out and a recoat every six weeks.

I have used this method for 20 years. The racks of the oven can be placed in the laundry tub when doing the washing. Use the soapy water to soak them with a little bi-carb. A steel pad rubbed down the rungs should remove all grease. I have passed this method on to some manufacturers who, after seeing the condition of my oven after many years, have recommended it to their customers.

Windows, glass and mirrors

A 'chamois' is an excellent investment. It is soft so will not scratch, nor does it leave streaks on the glass. Do not put it in very hot water, always lay it out to dry after use and it will last for years. Avoid window cleaning fluids as these encourage growth of mould on the glass or contain chemicals which may upset you. If the glass is very dirty, straight white vinegar on a sponge will do the trick. Rinse and finish off with chamois. (Do not use vinegar on chamois.) Warm water with a dash of methylated spirits is often used, but the vinegar will work just as well.

Deodorisers

Use a little lavender oil or dried flowers or herbs. Potpourri is pleasant, or use your own rose petals.

Vacuum-cleaning

Vacuum-cleaning can be very tiring. There is a theory that the motor itself has an adverse effect on debilitated people. However, if there is no kind person to perform this task for you, try a room at a time and use your mask if the carpet is relatively new. Dried herbs or flowers can be placed in the vacuum bag whilst cleaning to sweeten the air. Rosemary is lovely.

Polishes
Be careful with these. For silver and brass, bi-carb can be used although it is not 100 per cent effective. The fumes from most of the silver and brass cleaners will probably affect you so it is not worth the risk. Amway Metal Polish is promoted as being non-toxic. Mask and gloves should be worn.

For furniture, Nicholas Kiwi Pty Ltd who make Sheraton Teak oil say it has no formaldehyde or aromatic solvents although it does contain petrochemicals. I can tolerate it in small doses, however I recommend a mask should be worn. A safe alternative is beeswax softened on the stove and mixed with olive or light vegetable oil. Antique wax No 42 (made by Bio-Products) is excellent and has a pleasant aroma of lemon oil.

When I spoke to Nicholas Kiwi, I recommended that they should think seriously about non-petrochemical polishes. They were not averse to the idea at all as they do use some organic waxes. We will see what happens.

China Painting
If the smell of the gum turps used for mixing the paints is a problem, try olive oil instead. There is also a water-based medium available.

Glues
Aquadhere Wood-Working Glue and Semco Hobby Glue do not contain volatile solvents.

Candles
Greenpeace 7-hour candles made from non-toxic wax. These are available at health food stores, distributed by Whole Harvest Distributors (see Directory). 50 cents of the purchase

price goes to Greenpeace. These are lovely natural-looking candles.

Dealing with pests

Always read the labels on products, especially those which are designed to kill insects. Surface sprays, pest strips, cat and dog flea collars and cockroach baits should be treated with great caution. Some of these contain dichlorvos or chlorpyrifos. Be wary of any product which has the words 'Anti Cholinesterase' on the packaging. Rat poisons should also be treated with great caution. Investigate any poisons which you propose to use as many contain very harmful chemicals.

'Quassis chips', mentioned earlier as a treatment for head lice, can be sprinkled in roof cavities and will dissuade pests including possums.

Flies

A fly swat is essential. Bug-Off fly spray can be used sparingly if necessary. It is a mixture of natural oils mixed with 40 parts of water and is used in an atomiser. It is available at health food stores (ask them to get it in for you) and is made by the Natural Oil Workers Co-op (see Directory for address page 210).

Ants and cockroaches

Bug-Off is also excellent for these pests as cockroaches hate the smell and it does kill them as it contains pyrethrum oil. It smells strongly of eucalyptus, so wear a mask.

A mixture of borax (20 per cent) and honey (80 per cent) will also help. Place it in a lid and slide the lid under the refrigerator away from little hands. Ant-rid is similar and can be used in the same way. Bi-carb sprinkled on the area will also help to deter. Zoro Zoro Cockroach traps are excellent.

Fleas
Spray Bug-Off over the floor last thing at night and close off the room. Vacuum frequently and remember to empty the cleaner outside each time. Lavender oil is a good deterrent and a little mixed with water can be sprayed on carpet instead of Bug-Off. Crushed leaves of fennel is another deterrent as is a sprinkle of Epsom Salts.

An enterprising Sydney company, Sunotex Pty Ltd (see Directory page 210), has marketed a non-toxic flea trap. It is a metal tray with a light which attracts the fleas. Strips covered with a sticky substance trap the fleas. Available at Woolworths/Safeways.

Personal Insect Repellent
Bug-Off Personal Repellent is very effective, as is Sandy's Natural Insect Repellent distributed by Whole Harvest (see Directory). Available at health food stores. Use sparingly.

Moths and silverfish
Sunlight/Velvet laundry soap kept amongst clothes and linen is a deterrent, as is lavender oil or dried lavender. Eucalyptus or citronella oil is also effective. Epsom salts sprinkled in the corners of the cupboards assist. Make sure cupboards are cleaned out twice yearly if possible. Try some dried sage or tansy in wardrobes and pantry.

Bay leaves stored with grains and flours will repel weevils, moths and other insects.

• Do not use pest strips, napthalene or moth balls.

Outside

Pet care

Most dogs and cat flea collars contain dichlorvos (see Pesticides, herbicides and other toxic chemicals) but a range of non-toxic pet care products, distributed by Whole Harvest Distributors, is available at health food stores and some Woolworths/Safeways including Sandy's Flea Shampoo, Sandy's Flea Rinse, Sandy's Dog Flea Powder, Sandy's Cat Flea Powder, Sandy's Herbal Dog collar and Sandy's Herbal Cat collar.

Washing the dog

Use a bland soap — Herbon is excellent. Add a few drops of lavender oil to the last rinse, or rub in crushed fennel for fleas. Wormwood leaves made into tea make a good flea rinse. Avoid flea washes containing pesticides.

Gardening in general

Growing herbs and flowers in and around the vegetables is not only beneficial to the garden but also to us.

Marigolds and chrysanthemums as well as orange nasturtiums planted around the vegetable garden help to keep the pests at bay.

Basil and tansy will keep away flies and fruit fly. Garlic planted around roses will deter aphids, red spider in tomatoes and leaf curl.

Parsley and chives grow well together.

Parsley near tomatoes will deter aphids.

Geraniums planted around grapes will repel Japanese beetle.

Hyssop will deter cabbage moth, helps grape vines and makes an efficient spray for bacterial diseases.

Lavender is beneficial to garden and home.

Oregano is good amongst cabbages.

Pennyroyal will deter ants and, if rubbed on the skin, will deter mosquitoes.

Pepper sprinkled on damp leaves will deter caterpillars.

Grow rosemary and sage together near cabbages, but not potatoes.

Sage protects carrots.

Wormwood should be grown away from plants. However it's very good grown in the vicinity of fruit trees.

Grow borage amongst strawberries.

Chamomile helps other plants to grow and is beneficial to the compost heap.

Do not grow onions near peas or beans, they won't thrive.

Do not grow tomatoes near potatoes, they won't thrive.

A garlic spray can be made by putting 6 cloves garlic and a cup of water into the blender. Fine blend, strain through fine cotton or muslin, add half a teaspoon of Herbon detergent or pure soap, add one cup of water and place in atomiser. This is a very effective spray.

Spray cucumbers with nettle tea to cure and avoid mildew.

A few saucers or shallow dishes slightly depressed into the soil, filled with beer, will dispose of snails and slugs. Sand sprinkled around plants will deter them also.

We had a very unfortunate experience with snail pellets. Our next-door neighbour had inadvertently left the packet accessible to our dog who decided to breakfast on the pellets and died as a result. The vet told us that our dog was not the first to die in such a way. Apparently a base of bran is used to entice the snails and slugs and this is also enticing to some animals.

Also remember that the snails and slugs which are killed by the snail pellets and powders are also food to the lizards and birds and so a chain reaction can occur.

Quassia chips made up as for the head lice treatment can be used as an effective garden spray also — see page 134.

'Tahara' market a range of natural garden sprays, including a range using pyrethrum and garlic, Eucalyptus Insecticide and All Seasons Oil.

'Garden Friend' natural garlic concentrate is available also from nurseries.

Compost and manure are excellent fertilisers, as is seaweed. We collect several bags of seaweed from a lake on the mid-north coast each time we visit.

It's wise to remember, though, that over-fertilising can be just as harmful as under-fertilising. I keep a thick layer of seaweed on top of my vegetable garden which stops weeds and gradually mulches down to rich soil.

The remainder of my garden, which is mostly native plants and trees, I mulch with leaves and twigs and it needs no treatment whatsoever except a little water when very dry.

Swimming pools

An ionic water purifier is available from Aquamatics Pty Ltd (see Directory page 224). This purifier works through two electrodes of silver and copper which are fitted into the lid of the hair and lint trap. They are electrically charged at 24 volts which causes the positive electrode to electrolyse itself into the water in the ionic form of its constituent metals.

A small amount of sodium dichlor is necessary occasionally to remove any stains from the pool.

The unit works particularly well in pebble lined pools, but it cannot be fitted to new marble sheen or concrete finishes because of the highly alkaline materials of construction.

It is essential that the PH level of the pool be kept at 7.2 and the bi-carb at 90 to 100 ppm and that the pool be kept clean.

Barbecues

Barbecues are part of the 'Aussie' way of life. They are delicious and create a relaxed atmosphere socially. But be careful not to burn food and use wood or charcoal to create your fire. Do not use kerosene and never burn the styrene and plastic wrappings. These give off very toxic fumes.

Burning off

You will notice that garbage dumps do not allow 'burning-off' because of the toxicity of the fumes from burning rubbish, especially plastics; many local councils have banned backyard burning to cut down the pollution generally. Except for large tree loppings, which should be taken to the tip, most of the garden refuse can be composted, returning to nature that which is being taken out. (My husband shreds it with the lawnmower.)

Cleaning the car

Use a safe detergent — either Herbon or Caring or O.L.C. — or Sunlight/Velvet laundry soap. Do not stand the car on the driveway where the soap or detergent will wash into the drains even though these are safe detergents and non-pollutant. Rather, stand the car on the lawn where the water and suds will fulfill another purpose. O.L.C. seems preferable as a windscreen washer. Vinegar is also excellent in the windscreen wash. It is also good for cutting the grime off the car windows.

Car polishes are a problem as they all seem to be petrochemical based. Beeswax and vegetable oil, melted and blended until cool, may suffice.

Charcoal face masks

These have kindly been donated by 3M Australia Pty Ltd to the ME Society of New South Wales on an ongoing basis and are available from the Society in a pack of two for $6.00, which covers postage and handling and a donation to research. (See Directory page 205).

A grey mask is available for protection from dust and petrochemicals (organic vapours) and a blue mask is for chlorine and sulphur dioxide (acid gases). Should the foam irritate the nose, stitch a small piece of fine cotton over it.

The home medicine chest

Homoeopathic First Aid Kit and Bach Flower Remedies from Martin and Pleasance (see Directory).
Vitamins and Minerals of choice.

Ointments and lotions

Health food stores stock a range of herbal ointments which are a must for the many accidents, bites, rashes, bruises etc.

which befall the average person. Arnica and Calendula are invaluable. The following list of ointments is supplied by Martin and Pleasance (see Directory). Their ointments are formulated in a non-greasy base and they also supply Arnica and Calendula Lotions. Ask your health food store to get them in.

Arnica

Arnica has been used throughout history as one of the best herbs for the healing of bruises and sprains. It may be used externally for all forms of inflammation but is not recommended for use on broken skin or open wounds. Apply three to four times daily.

Burn Cream

This cream contains Urtica Urens, Calendula and Hamamelis herbs which are traditionally of use in reducing inflammation and promoting healing of minor burns. Apply three to four times daily or as necessary. Seek medical attention for deep burns or signs of infection.

Calendula

Calendula is a herb reputed for treating inflammation of the skin due to minor infection or abrasions. It can be applied to bruises, sprains, scalds, minor burns and slow healing wounds such as skin ulcers. Apply to affected areas three times daily or as necessary.

Cutine Wet

Cutine wet is recommended for the treatment of eczema, psoriasis, ringworm and itchy, cracked skin conditions. Apply three times daily or as necessary.

Hamamelis

Hamamelis herb has a reputation for its astringent and soothing properties. It may be used in the treatment of bruises, painful inflammatory skin conditions or applied to varicose veins.

Hydrastis

Hydrastis is a herb reputed for its relief of skin conditions such as eczema, ringworm and pruritis (itching). Apply three times daily or as necessary.

Hypercal

Hypercal cream contains Calendula and Hypericum herbs which have been used traditionally to promote healing and relieve the pain of cuts, minor wounds and bruising. Apply three times daily.

Hypericum

Hypericum has a traditional use as being a valuable healing and anti-inflammatory herb. It has been used successfully in the treatment of wounds, bruises and minor burns.

Rescue Remedy Cream

This cream is prepared from a special combination of flower essences. Dr Bach used these flower essences externally on ulcers, lacerations, sprains, stings and minor burns. Apply when necessary.

Tea Tree

Tea tree is renowned for its antiseptic properties and is reputed to promote healing when applied to boils, acne, ringworm, cuts, scratches and insect bites. Apply three times daily.

Thuja

Thuja is a herb used as a treatment for warts and is reputed to be effective when applied externally for the treatment of ringworm and thrush. Apply two or three times daily.

Urtica Urens (nettle)
Urtica is a herb that has a reputation for its use in all forms of itchy skin conditions. It may be used on eczema of all types including childhood and nervous eczema. Apply three times daily.

Two other brands of Arnica Ointment are Herb of Life and Nature Spirit Herbal Products both of New South Wales (see Directory page 204). Arnica Massage Oil by Weleda (see Directory page 210) is excellent.

Newton's Pharmacy of Sydney (see Directory page 204) will make up herbal ointments, lotions and remedies. Make sure petroleum jelly is not the base for the ointments and check whether the lanoline is pesticide free. Australia-wide mail order service.

Cholesterol combatant

For anyone who has a cholesterol problem, Martin and Pleasance are marketing 'Lecipur A', available from health food stores. This product has undergone extensive clinical trials overseas during the last five years and has been clearly shown to be effective in reducing levels of Low Density Lipoprotein (those dangerous to health) and increasing or maintaining levels of High Density Lipoprotein (those deemed beneficial to health).

No side effects were noted.

This is a product derived from pure lecithin and reduces dangerous cholesterol by a natural safe method.

Olive oil

Olive oil has so many uses. As a body moisturiser, for fungus skin infections, used for cooking, taken for thrush/candida and used in making your cosmetics. It contains no cholesterol. It is also most useful as a lubricant of the anus and will help to prevent haemorrhoids; if a small amount of tissue starts to protrude, gently push it back using olive oil. I have been using olive oil for this purpose for years, and so far, despite having three children, including twins, I have no haemorrhoid problems. Olive oil is great for fungus infections, especially on the feet, and a few drops of tea tree oil added makes a great foot massage oil.

Tea tree oil

Tea Tree oil is an antiseptic distilled from the leaves of the paperbark tree, and is most effective as a germicidal and fungicidal. This warm, penetrating oil helps to promote healing, relieve pain and refurbish cut and bruised areas. It is used as a douche in the treatment of thrush/candida and can be taken in very small doses (two drops only to a maximum of ten drops per day) internally. It can be added to a mouthwash or gargle, makes the bathroom and toilet smell nice, and repels insects. It is also good on insect bites.

Eucalyptus oil

Eucalyptus oil is a wonderful antiseptic. It is bacteriostatic and antifungal. It can be used to repel insects, rinse woollens, disinfect the toilet and remove stains. If you have problems with salicylates, eucalyptus may not be tolerated.

Lavender oil

A few drops added to olive oil makes a refreshing and therapeutic massage oil.

Evening Primrose oil

Evening Primrose oil is derived from the seeds of the Evening Primrose.

Vita Glow market 'Efamol Marine' soft gelatin capsules combining Evening Primrose oil and fish oil and have conducted a series of tests on patients with ME/CFS in the UK. Although these results have not as yet been published, members of the ME Society have taken this product with advantageous results, and it has been found to be particularly effective in those patients who experience palpitations. The product is available at health food stores and chemists, but it is always wise to discuss taking a new preparation with your doctor before you do. There are no side effects other than occasional nausea, indigestion and headache.

A word of warning. The product 'Efamol Marine' is not to be taken by anyone with a history of epilepsy or schizophrenia, or by anyone on medication relating to those diseases, or anyone who has heavy periods.

Toiletries and Cosmetics

As this book goes to print the Federal Government has announced that all cosmetics must have the ingredients displayed on the packaging. This will make our individual allergies and preferences much easier to deal with in the ensuing years.

Soap

I would recommend Herbon Botanical Soap and Baby Soap, Caring Body Soap, Brot Bodyline Soap, Herbon Liquid Soap on Tap (pumps and refills), Sunlight/Velvet laundry soap and Simple Soap (available from chemists).

There is also a bland, unperfumed soap, which comes unwrapped, based on natural vegetable oils. It's distributed by Whole Harvest and is available from health food stores.

Personal Deodorant

Anti-perspirant deodorants generally contain aluminium and our bodies were designed to perspire to rid us of toxins. An alternative is Herb Valley made by Natural Product Distributors (see Directory page 210) and available from health food stores. Herbon, Caring and Weleda also manufacture deodorants. These are herbal and aluminium free. Herbon deodorant is perfume free.

Toothpaste
Weleda make Herbal Toothpaste and Plant Gel Toothpaste but Blackmores Herbal and Mineral Toothpaste is less expensive than the others and is excellent. A mixture of salt and bicarb is a cheap alternative — flavour with a few drops of peppermint oil.

Blackmores products are generally of a very high quality. But, being an old, established company, they still use petroleum jelly (vaseline) as a base for some of their ointments and there were traces of formaldehyde in some of their products. Their Product Development Manager has informed me that they are taking another close look at all their products and have ceased to purchase the ingredients which contained traces of formaldehyde. However some preservatives are 'formaldehyde donors' — although they do not contain formaldehyde as such, they form formaldehyde in the product and in so reacting, destroy bacteria. The question of perfumes, some of which are synthesised from petroleum products, is also being assessed.

Blackmores are working towards systems which lead to the elimination of substances causing sensitivities and towards more effective natural preservatives. This is indeed a very responsible attitude.

Hair Care
Hairdressing salons can be a real problem to ME/CFS sufferers. The perming solution, the shampoos, the holding sprays and gels are in the main intolerable. Try to get an appointment at the beginning of the day before the perming takes place and take your own shampoo. If a hairdresser will call at your home, that is the answer. I do not recommend perms if you suffer ME/CFS.

I do recommend Herbon Ginseng Shampoo or Anti-dandruff Shampoo and Conditioner, Blackmores Chamomile

Conditioner and Golden Wattle (Bee Pollen) Shampoo and Conditioner. (Melrose Lab. See Directory page 210.)

Also Brot Bodyline Shampoo Bar and Weleda range of shampoos and conditioner, as well as Caring shampoos and conditioner. From the chemist, Simple Shampoo.

These shampoos are petrochemical and formaldehyde free.

Coconut oil massaged into the scalp is excellent for dry hair and, mixed with a couple of drops of Tea Tree oil, is good for dandruff and any irritations of the scalp.

Lemon juice is very good for oily hair — add one tablespoon of strained juice to a jug of warm water for the last rinse. It will lighten fair hair slightly.

Beer gives the hair body and can be used as a last rinse.

Chamomile tea is good for fair hair, as a last rinse.

A hairspray can be made as follows: cut one lemon into pieces, boil the pieces in one cup of water until liquid is reduced to almost half, strain through gauze or fine cotton. Add a few drops of alcohol (vodka) to preserve and pour into a spray bottle. BWC (Beauty Without Cruelty) Hairspray is recommended. (Melrose. See Directory.)

Shaving Cream

Weleda Shaving Creme made from natural oils.

After Shave

Witch-hazel, available from health food stores and some chemists is excellent as is Weleda Shaving Lotion. Bavarian by Nutri-metics is just tolerable.

Weleda products are made from bio-dynamically grown plants, all natural ingredients and are designed to have a positive benefit to the skin. The range is extensive and includes skin and beauty therapy, skin care products, dental care and mouth hygiene, shampoos and conditioner, massage preparations, baby preparations and shaving requisites. They are available at health food stores (ask the manager to get them in — address in Directory). Their packaging is environmentally-friendly.

Handcreams and moisturisers

Nature's Gate moisturising lotion, Millcreek Moisturiser, Weleda Hand Care Gel. See pages 172-4 for further moisturing products.

Sun protection and sunscreens

These I have not found entirely satisfactory. They either burn my skin, or I cannot stand the smell. Some of the chemicals which prevent sunburn are now thought to cause skin cancers. It seems we just can't win. I am not totally comfortable with any of them except zinc cream which is messy. (My dermatologist tells me this is the best.)

Try not to expose your skin to the sun and always wear a hat and sunglasses (polaroid) to filter out the ultraviolet rays. When fishing I wear long cotton pants, a long-sleeved shirt and gloves with the fingers cut off, plus of course sunglasses and a hat. Be particularly careful with children. Do not expose them to the sun. It is during the tender years that the skin cancers of the future are formed. Again, be careful what you put on tender skin. Remember that we absorb harmful chemicals through the pores. Millcreek Waterproof SPF 15 Sunblock (unperfumed) is used by myself and my family as well as some of my friends with satisfaction. I am now suffering from exposure to the sun (from sunbaking when younger) and I have had several skin cancers removed.

Sunburn

Aloe Vera, cold tea and witch-hazel will all relieve sunburn. Aloe Vera is excellent. If you have the plant in your garden, cut a leaf, peel back the flesh and use the colourless egg-white type sap to cover the burnt area. Keep the skin as cool as possible.

Burn Cream from Martin and Pleasance (address in Directory) is an excellent cream to keep in the house. If your health food store does not have it in stock ask them to order it in.

Talcum powder

I cannot find an unperfumed talc on the market. Simple talc is not marketed in Australia at present. I did approach Blackmores who told me that talc is not good for the skin as it clogs the pores and therefore they are loathe to produce it. However, Weleda do make Calendula Baby Talc.

Toilet tissues

Why not use old-fashioned handkerchiefs? If we do, we are not consuming and throwing away, not exposing ourselves to dioxin or formaldehyde, and we are helping to save our trees.

Toilet paper

Buy only unbleached, unperfumed paper. Use very sparingly. Available from some health food stores, Woolworths, Coles and Franklins.

Tampons and pads

Remember the people who were getting sick from the tampons? A safe (reusable) alternative is 'natural sponge'. This can be purchased from chemist shops and cut to size to make a reusable tampon. Moisten with purified water before use, wash thoroughly with bland soap and water, add a couple of drops of tea tree oil to the rinse and you will have a safe alternative and save money.

I experienced rashes and soreness with deodorised pads so be careful with these. Although they were bleached, 'No Frills' were the least upsetting to myself. A piece of clean sheeting placed over the pad should protect you if you are sensitive. A friend uses 'Sure & Natural' with success. When I was young these products did not exist.

There is need for unbleached sanitary pads and cloth re-usable, washable pads for those who are really environmentally conscious.

Baby products

Use only natural oils — olive, avocado, almond, apricot etc. Available from health food stores. Do not use baby oil (most are based on mineral — petrochemical — oils) on either yourself or children.

Zinc and castor oil cream is good for nappy rash but I'd advise you to investigate the other ingredients. I have used McGloin's available from chemist stores. Blackmores cold pressed apricot oil is also extremely effective for nappy rash in babies and children. Weleda Baby Cream, Lotion, Talc, Oil and Soap are recommended.

As some of the baby shampoos contain petrochemicals and formaldehyde, it is much safer to use only the mildest of baby soap. Herbon and Brot Bodyline are excellent.

I had a long chat with several very helpful representatives from Johnson & Johnson Australia Pty Ltd who informed me that, with my petrochemical and formaldehyde problems, except for Baby Soap and Powder their products would not be suitable. They were kind enough to give me detailed product information, however they have since requested that I do not publish this information. I shall comply with their request.

Johnson's Baby Soap and Baby Powder are petrochemical and formaldehyde free in formulation, however, they were unable to give me information regarding the perfume which I, personally, cannot tolerate.

I did appreciate the trouble Johnson & Johnson went to on my behalf. If any further product information is required, may I suggest that a telephone call to Johnson & Johnson should clarify the matter.

Avoid disposable nappies which are chlorine bleached. Some Huggies are non-chlorine-bleached. Old-fashioned cloth nappies washed in Herbon or Sunlight/Velvet are by far the best. All bleached paper has a small content of dioxin and disposable nappies are causing pollution.

Eye makeup

Nutri-metics have a range of unperfumed eye creams made from cocoa butter. Their mascara is water-based and tolerated by myself if used occasionally. Many of their other products are too heavily perfumed for me.

Perfumes

In the main, perfumes should be avoided as many contain toluene or phenol. The eau-de-colognes and toilette waters like 4711 and lavender water are acceptable but be aware that even natural perfumes like jasmine, wisteria, jonquils and gardenias are not well tolerated by people with petrochemical sensitivities as they contain natural terpenes.

There is a range of natural perfume oils at most health food stores. Choose one to suit.

Nail polish

I would not recommend using this product at all. It often contains formaldehyde and the fumes from the acetone are toxic. If you must use it, make sure you use it outside in the fresh air, and use your mask.

Yves Rocher, who specialise in herbal cosmetics, do make nail polishes. Maybe they are not so toxic. I have not tried them.

Lipstick

Although many brands of lipstick are made from mostly natural ingredients, the preservatives and perfumes are a problem to many people, including myself.

The Nutri-metics range of lipstick are made from cocoa butter but I cannot tolerate the perfumes nor the taste. The Yves Rocher range uses only natural ingredients and I *can* tolerate their lipstick which tastes like strawberry syrup. There are many people with allergies who cannot find a suitable lipstick and I must say that when I was very ill I experienced much more sensitivity than I do now.

A last resort and safe alternative is beetroot juice. Use a juice extractor or put the raw beetroot into a blender and then strain through a fine strainer or piece of fine cotton material. Add a few drops of vodka or a little vinegar to preserve and keep in the refrigerator. Use on lips and cover with lip ointment (see 'Facial and body treatments') to retain colour and give a glossy look. My lip ointment, made to a firmer consistency by adding more beeswax, can be coloured with cochineal or beetroot juice. Just mix a very small quantity in an egg cup and keep in the refrigerator. *Do be careful* with artificial red colouring — test it first on your wrist to make sure it is tolerable and use it only as a last resort.

Time permitting, a good deal of fun can be had by experimenting with cosmetics, ointments and lotions, using only everyday ingredients. Cocoa butter, if procurable, is a good base for lipstick. Remember that the shelf-life of homemade cosmetics is limited.

I have tried some of the Yves Rocher range of cosmetics and apart from the lipstick had difficulty with many of them. The company kindly sent me a couple of samples of their 'Florilia 2' (cleanser, toner and day cream) but the perfume 'knocked me out'. Some of their soaps were interesting and they do advertise that they use only natural ingredients. Their products are quite strongly perfumed. They have direct selling offices in each state of Australia.

I investigated the 'Body Shop' range of cosmetics which are in the main perfumed and I could not tolerate them. However, they have made a real effort to produce natural cosmetics, although I do wish manufacturers would realise that not everyone likes perfumes. The products do contain small amounts of preservatives and lanoline. Their unperfumed soaps look very interesting and their refills and packaging are environmentally-friendly.

Simple products

The best are Simple Soap, Clear Soap, Skin Tonic, Facial Mask, Facial Scrub, Shampoos and Hair Conditioner. They do not contain perfume or formaldehyde and are petrochemical-free. Their other products contain a small quantity of mineral oil and their deodorant contains aluminium as the anti-perspirant.

The distributors are Smith & Nephew (Australia) Pty Ltd and they are available in chemists.

Facial and body treatments

Here are a couple of treatments I have been using for years. A quarter of a cup of milk mixed with half a teaspoon of honey makes a marvellous facial. I often wash my face with milk, buttermilk or yogurt and leave on overnight. Avoid very hot or very cold liquids on face otherwise veins may show on cheeks.

White of egg will tighten the skin, so if you wish to look younger for the evening, this is a trick used by the movie stars. Save for a special occasion!

Lemon juice is a great cleanser on oily parts of the face and, mixed with almond or olive oil, is good on the hands. Wheat germ oil is an excellent moisturiser (so long as you don't have a wheat allergy).

If the eyes are tired, lie down, close eyes, place cucumber slices over them. A few drops of cucumber juice in the eyes will rejuvenate them. If eyes are sore, bathe in warm boiled water with a little salt added. Salt and water is very soothing to mucous membranes. Chamomile teabags are good too.

Teenage acne can be a real problem. Keeping the skin and hair super clean is very important. Use honey and milk to draw out pimples and lemon as a cleanser on the oily spots. Most teenagers eventually grow out of the problem, once the hormones settle down (by the time they are 18-20). Those who have a really chronic problem should consult a specialist in this field as they could have a problem with the actual pores of the skin. Witch-hazel is an excellent astringent.

Wheatgerm, almond or apricot oil makes a good moisturiser after bathing and I use wheat germ oil on my face and hands.

Remember my mentioning that when I was using a lanoline-based calendula ointment my lips broke out in sores which defied identification in pathology tests. Here is my recipe for the lip salve which I have used ever since. The cod liver oil was added to heal up the sores so if the slightly fishy smell worries you, omit it and make up the quantity with olive oil. Use calendula concentrate instead. However, cod liver oil has excellent healing qualities.

> 1/2 cup of olive oil
> 1 tablespoon cod liver oil
> 1 tablespoon wheat germ oil
> 2 crushed zinc tablets (powdered)
> 10 drops Tea Tree oil
> 30g (1oz) beeswax (generous)
> 30 drops calendula concentrate (optional)

Heat all ingredients on stove until beeswax has melted, stir thoroughly. Test a few drops on a cold plate to see if the mixture solidifies to an ointment consistency. It needs to be a firm consistency, much the same as lipstick. The hardness of the beeswax affects the consistency. If you find it is not hard enough, just too oily, reheat the ingredients and add just a little more beeswax.

Try to purchase cold pressed oils. For those who have wheat allergies substitute the wheat germ oil with apricot or other oil of choice.

Pour mixture into small jars. Save small glass jars which contained vitamins etc. for this purpose. Baby food jars are also good, especially the ones with the wide tops. The above mixture will fill 3–4 small vitamin jars.

Cosmetics — in summary

For those who are extremely sensitive to commercially produced cosmetics, stick with the natural cold pressed oils as moisturisers. Wheat germ oil is very light, rich in Vitamin E and is a wonderful moisturiser. Use only the ingredients from your cupboard and refrigerator for skin care and general body care together with a pure soap for cleansing.

I recommend: Blanca's Natural Products which offer a range of moderately-priced cleansers, toners, moisturisers, cell repairers, de-pigmentation creams and products for the aging. They're available from The Women's Advisory Service (see Directory page 208). These products have been specially formulated for people with sensitivities and are unperfumed.

Dr Hauschka Cosmetics are exceptional, but the prices are as well — these are definitely up-market cosmetics! The range is extensive and covers body oils, coloured day creams, eyelid tone, lip and cheek shade and a range of skin care products. They are truly natural products with no preservatives. The Australian distributors are Helios Enterprises Limited (see Directory page 208).

I would recommend reading *Herbal Cosmetics* by Camilla Hepper which I obtained from my health food store. It is an English publication and although some of the ingredients may not be available here, it will give you clues and recipes to make your own cosmetics and you can use your own imagination to improvise with flowers which grow here. It is distributed by Collins and should be available through anyone who has an account with them including newsagents and health food stores.

Feed Your Face by Dian Buchman is an excellent book as well, full of treatments made from basic products in the pantry and refrigerator. Unfortunately it is only available at a few libraries.

Foods, cooking, packaging and storage

Foods to avoid

If possible, do not consume processed foods, fast foods, foods with artificial preservatives and additives, foods and oils in plastic containers, drinks in aluminium cans, milk and drinks in plastic containers and cardboard cartons, tinned foods, packet soups, wines and beer (unless produced without preservatives e.g. Cooper's) and bleached flour. Always read the labels and buy a copy of *The New Additive Code Breaker* as mentioned previously.

There is a move afoot by the large food manufacturers to persuade the government not to require that the ingredients (including additives) be put on the packaging, and to relax the laws with regard to the percentage of meat etc, in particular foods, including sausages and devon. (Their complaint is that it is an expensive exercise!) Do not let this happen: write to your local member. We all need to know just what is contained in the food we eat.

Milk and milk products

It is a shame that we have mostly dispensed with glass packaging for milk products. As researched and stated later in this chapter many plastic containers leach plasticisers and other chemicals into foods, especially fatty foods. Plastic milk containers are a pollution problem and cardboard milk cartons, although they are presently being modified, are lined with plastic. Trees are needed for the production of milk cartons and cartons cannot be recycled. Why have we changed our packaging when glass is so good? Is it just the whim of the supermarkets who prefer cardboard and plastic because they are not heavy and do not break? Surely our health and the environment should come first.

No-one can dispute the fact that milk tastes so much better

in glass bottles. There was an overwhelming response to this when the problem was discussed on Radio 2BL in Sydney. So many people complained that they could not buy milk in glass. Glass can be re-cycled.

Butter, cream and cheese

From organic and bio-dynamic farms, these are available from some health food stores and suppliers of organic produce, including Russells and Chem-free Meats of Sydney (See Directory). Keep asking. Margarine is not recommended.

Beverages

An Australian tea, from Madura Tea Estates Pty Ltd is free of any pesticides, although the tea plantation does use artificial fertilisers.

However tea and coffee should be used very sparingly. If taking homoeopathic medicines, coffee is not permitted. Herbal teas are much more beneficial. Chamomile, verbena, lemon grass and rose hip are just a few of the many herbal teas available and dandelion coffee is pleasant and beneficial.

Lots of pure water cannot be bettered. Mineral water should be taken sparingly.

Drinks which contain preservatives should be avoided.

Freshly squeezed fruit juices are preferable but they should be diluted.

'Norfolk Punch' is very new on the market and is a delightful blend of herbs. It is still made according to an original Benedictine monks' recipe, using the well water (which contains selenium) on site in Norfolk, United Kingdom and strict adherence to the organic method of growing the herbs and other ingredients has been maintained. It is non-alcoholic, can be drunk hot or cold and is delicious. It appears to have therapeutic qualities and taken at bedtime induces sound sleep. It can be purchased at health food stores throughout Australia.

It is marketed by the Colonial Beverage Company who will

be pleased to hear from anyone having difficulties procuring it (see Directory page 210).

Alcoholic drinks are usually not well tolerated by ME/CFS sufferers. However for those interested there is a range of inexpensive, organically grown, preservative-free meads and wines available from Mount Vincent Mead and a red wine from Botobolar Vineyard Pty Ltd, both of Mudgee, New South Wales. These vineyards will take mail and telephone orders for delivery throughout Australia (see Directory).

Organically grown grains

The 'Demeter' range is available from health food stores, and includes a wide range of breads and flours, rolled oats, grains and kernels, breadcrumbs, toasted muesli, noodles, whole grain pastries, whole grain pies and quiches, yeast-free and sugar-free pastries, whole grain biscuits and grape juice.

'Demeter' bio-dynamic produce is grown by an advanced organic method, applying Rudolf Steiner's agricultural indications, which strive to bring healing to the earth and human beings. No artificial fertilisers, pesticides or chemical additives are used at any stage of growing, storage and production.

'Demeter' products are presently only available in New South Wales — Central Coast, South Coast, Canberra and Blue Mountains. However, they will supply interstate upon request. Available from Helios Enterprises Ltd, (see Directory page 209).

Baking Powder

Low Allergy Baking Powder (Aluminium Free) is made by Robins Wholefood Kitchen, South Australia (see Directory page 211). Use 1 teaspoon per half cup of flour. Available from health food stores.

Other foods

Many other foods are available from health food stores: a

range of 'real culture' yogurt, including Bornhoffen cow's milk and Carnochan goat's milk yogurt; soy milk and tofu; soy sauce, with or without wheat, packed in glass; vegetable oils, packed in glass; freshly made peanut butter; natural honeys; dried fruits, organically grown and sun dried; nuts; organically grown grains and flours; freshly baked breads, as well as 'Demeter', including 'Dallas' a new bakery from Northbridge, New South Wales; fruit juices; and purified water. Some are now stocking fresh fruit and vegetables.

Organically grown produce

A comprehensive list of suppliers of organically grown grains, flours, fruit and vegetables, meat etc. throughout Australia and appears on page 211--223 of the Directory.

Storage of food

The plastic age is a problem. We should all be demanding glass packaging and a minimum of unbleached paper wrapping so that it can be recycled.

There are a variety of glass storage containers on the market and although they have plastic lids, so long as the food does not touch the lids, it should be safe. The CSIRO confirmed that chemicals leach into food from plastic containers and the gentleman I spoke to there agreed that we should all be 'going for glass' as it was the safest and could be recycled.

Coles Stores sell glass storage containers and there are more expensive ones available at kitchen shops and department stores. I use screw top jars of varying sizes to great advantage. They do not take up much room and the contents are visible. Pyrex, corning ware and crockery casserole dishes with lids can be used to store larger items.

I always use greaseproof paper to wrap sandwiches. It is not wise to put plastic film directly onto food.

Plastic ice-cream containers should not be used to store foods, especially hot foods, and should never be used for cooking in the microwave oven.

After exhaustive inquiries from various manufacturers including Glad Wrap and OSO, and from the CSIRO and the National Health and Medical Research Council, there seem to be a large number of questions unanswered. In September 1987 *CHOICE* magazine published a report on pre-wrapped cheese and meat packed 'in-house' by some supermarkets. All of the stores were using PVC film wrap and tests were conducted on meat and cheese products to establish whether the cancer-linked chemicals di-octyl adipate (DOA) and di-octyl phthalate (DOP) had leached into the foods. They reported ' ... small quantities of DOA in most of the foods and in two of the cheeses we found DIOP — chemically very similar to DOP.' As it is very difficult to tell the difference between polyethylene film and the PVC film consumers should be wary and ask their supermarket.

The problem of leaching has been borne out by one of the manufacturers of plastic food packaging who has recommended that people like myself, who are chemically sensitive, keep the use of plastic food packaging to a minimum. They further state the effects upon any individual of any additives present will depend presumably not only on the type and concentration of the additive but also the extent to which it might be released from the plastic and the susceptibility of that individual to the particular material.

They also state that they do not know the exact composition of some of the materials they use as they come from Japan and are proprietory information. Also there may be none or perhaps up to 4 or 5 anti-oxidants or other aids involved in the processing of a particular resin into an end-product. Very often raw material suppliers treat their additive packages as proprietory information and do not disclose it to the manufacturer.

I do thank this particular manufacturer for being so honest about the fact that various chemicals *do* leach into our food from plastic containers and packaging.

The CSIRO indicated to me that polyethylene, which has no plasticisers and is used extensively for food containers as well as film wrap and bags, is manufactured to Australian Standard 2070 which does include specified miscellaneous additives including antioxidants BHT (butylated hydroxytoluene) and BHA (butylated hydroxyanisole). Neither are recommended for children.

The National Health and Medical Research Council sent me a 'Summary of Data Reported and Evaluation' of BHT. No data was available to evaluate the carcinogenicity of BHT to humans. 'There was limited evidence of carcinogenicity ... in experimental animals.'

According to *The New Additive Code Breaker*, BHA and BHT can leach from polyethylene film. However, it is difficult to find out which manufacturers are adding BHT or any of the other miscellaneous additives. Fatty foods and oils will attract plasticisers, however other chemicals can leach into food, depending on the type of food stored, according to information I was given by one scientist.

The two representatives I spoke to from GLAD Products were very helpful. Their film wrap, garbage and freezer bags are made from polyethylene which contains no plasticisers. However, Glad Microwave oven wrap is made from polyvinylidene chloride (PVDC). This product includes the plasticiser di-n-hexylazelate. The product came upon the market just after *CHOICE* had performed their tests and therefore they were not looking for this particular plasticiser and do not know whether it leaches out.

OSO brand of film and bags are made from polyethylene. According to their representative they do not market any PVC or PVDC products.

There are numerous brands of plastic bags and film wrap on the market. Many do not say what they are made from and various brands vary from state to state as to their contents. My only advice then is to read the packaging and if there is insufficient information, phone the manufacturer or the distributor.

Efforts are being made to make plastic bags biodegradable. GLAD Products are in the process of bringing out garbage bags which will degrade in soil as cornstarch is added to the formula thus encouraging bacteria to attack the product and break it down.

The plastics industry seems to me to be a Pandora's box of possible problems, both in the manufacturing processes and in the effects on our environment. There does not seem to be enough known about the effects on our health. As has been the case in the past, it often takes many years for the harmful effects to become evident, therefore my personal opinion is 'when in doubt — don't'. Glass is a tried and proven, safe receptacle for food. Glass can be re-cycled. Food tastes better in glass. It is all a matter of supply and demand. If you prefer glass packaging and unbleached wrapping paper — write and ask for it!

I try to avoid plastic packaging, especially with food, as much as humanly possible. I can no longer purchase glass bottles of vegetable oils, other than olive oil, at my supermarkets. However, they are available at health food stores. I have milk delivered in bottles to my door and only wish that yogurt and cream were similarly packaged.

As far as frozen food is concerned, I purchase only fresh food. Meat can be wrapped fresh in greaseproof paper (I will feel much happier when chlorine bleaching has ceased) and then placed in cellophane bags which are biodegradable. It can be frozen in this fashion.

(Incidentally, Woolworths cut cheese for me from their large blocks and wrap it in paper. We only have to ask!)

My vegetables and fruit (organically grown) are packed in brown paper bags, placed in a cardboard box which I return, and delivered to my door.

Greaseproof paper
OSO referred me to Caxton Paper when I made inquiries.

All greaseproof paper is imported into Australia. This was confirmed by Australian Paper Mills. At present greaseproof paper marketed in Australia is semi-bleached with chlorine. However, Caxton Paper (New Zealand) are in the process of changing to hydrogen peroxide as the bleaching agent. This will not create dioxin in the manufacturing process. When I inquired why they could not produce 'unbleached' greaseproof paper I was told that they had just set up a new plant in New Zealand and that the production of unbleached paper would require very extensive and expensive changes to the plant.

Greaseproof paper is also imported from Scandinavia. As European countries have become very conscious of the problems caused by chlorine bleaching, I am sure it will not be long before we can get unbleached greaseproof paper from this source. I must say it is encouraging to see that manufacturers are taking up the challenge of protecting us and our environment.

'Cellophane' film

'Cellophane' is made from wood but the film made to store food is coated with PVDC 2%. The film is applied with either water or solvent. 'Cellophane' is biodegradable and many organically grown products, including 'Demeter' are packed in cellophane.

The following information was obtained from ACL Films.

'Cellophane' is a natural product. It is produced from wood pulp manufactured from eucalyptus tree plantations that are farmed. The trees are cut down but do not die. They soon send out new shoots that mature in three years to a size ready to be harvested again. Farming in this manner does not denude whole forests.

Cellulose film is probably the most benign of all packaging films in use today. Those grades of cellulose film used in direct contact with food are approved for this application by the Federal Drug Agency of the USA and other similarly strong agencies in Germany and Japan. Cellophane is biodegradable, does not pollute and is not known to cause allergies.

'Cellophane' bags are not retailed as this goes to print but I have purchased a quantity, size 26cm x 47 cm (10 1/2" x 18 1/2") which will be available in bundles of 50 for $6.00 or $12.00 for 100, plus $4.50 for postage in New South Wales and $6.50 for other states. Prices subject to change. Please write to me at the address given in the Directory on page 211. 'Cellophane' bags can be wiped out and re-used.

Cooking

The best saucepans are those by Crown Corning 'Vision' glass. Stainless steel and cast iron are also good. Avoid teflon coated pans and aluminium cookware. Use pyrex, china or crockery in the microwave. A dessert bowl with a glass saucepan lid is great for small items.

Choose electricity rather than gas for cooking. Gas fumes are toxic.

Vegetables are better steamed or stir-fried, not overcooked. Never reuse cooking oils.

Plastic electric jugs and kettles are not recommended.

Other sources of toxicity

Refuelling the car

Do not inhale petrol fumes. It is far better to go to a service station which gives full service. If this is impossible, stand 'up wind' of the tank and wear your mask. Avoid contact with the skin.

New vehicles can be a problem with the interior vinyl and plastics 'blowing out'. Make sure to not leave the vehicle in the sun and then get in without airing it off. Never allow anyone to smoke in your car.

When travelling, do not sit behind a vehicle with the windows open so that you are inhaling all the fumes from the vehicle in front. Carbon monoxide is poisonous. Rather, seal the car up in thick traffic and air it off later. I have installed a fan in the back of my car which circulates the interior air. An air conditioner will do the same on recycle. I nearly drive my husband mad when we are travelling but anything is better than becoming ill. A mask is a must for those impossible situations.

Air conditioning

Air conditioning can be another problem when it comes to indoor air pollution. The 'new building sickness syndrome' has been much talked about. Obviously many people are affected by the fumes blowing out of new building materials, plastics, carpets and paints, many of which contain extremely toxic chemicals. If there is not the provision for proper ventilation (open windows), it can take a long time for these fumes to be expelled from the building — in the meantime, the inhabitants of the building are absorbing and building up toxins in their bodies.

Pest treatments, other toxins, cigarette smoke and bacteria can also be recycled through the air conditioning systems, depending on the type of air conditioner installed.

I find it impossible to visit some large air conditioned hospitals for this very reason, whereas I have no problems with the Royal Women's in Paddington, Sydney or the Mater in North Sydney where there are open windows and fresh air circulating all the time. Neither of these hospitals reek of disinfectant and anaesthetics as soon as I reach the door.

Heating

Solar heating has been perfected for water heating but has, as yet, to be perfected for efficient home heating purposes. There are solar heating panels available and the technology is improving all the time — it must be an answer for the future.

Reverse-cycle air conditioners are the most economical form of electrical heating but be sure to clean the filter frequently as you can get a build-up of mould, especially after the summer months when you have been cooling the house. There are other forms of electrical heating that are non-pollutant but they are much more expensive. (The pollution caused by the production of electricity is a problem we need to solve urgently.)

A wood burning combustion heater is efficient and economical, and does not put smoke into the house, however, it does cause pollution even though it burns very slowly. (see under 'How we can start to clean up our world' pages 188–98.)

An open fire burns a great amount of wood and produces much more smoke, both inside and outside the home, thus creating pollution. Many people are allergic to the smoke from burning wood.

Coal and coke fires are a definite 'no-no' because of the pollution.

Avoid gas heaters, particularly unflued, free-standing heaters. Avoid oil heaters as these sometimes cause fumes in the house and certainly cause fumes outside the house.

Conclusion

The Effect of ME/CFS on my life

ME/CFS has changed my way of life completely, and I must say it is for the better. I have been introduced to a different form of medicine which will benefit myself and family for the rest of our lives and I have made many new friends. My sickness has also influenced my family who have become so much more aware of the toxic drugs and chemicals in our environment and they avoid them as much as possible. It has made us realise that we can live very happily and comfortably *without* the many toxic products flashed on the TV screen day after day. It has made us all conscious of what we are doing to our world.

It has influenced the lives of people who know me, and particularly many people on the mid-north coast where pesticide and herbicide spraying is a way of life. My neighbours and friends are so much more conscious of the devastating effects these chemicals can have as they have watched me through the various stages of my sickness, and I must say I looked and felt pretty ghastly. They watched me trying to walk — I was like an old woman — and it has really set them thinking. No-one around me sprays any more with toxic chemicals, and after threatening to sue the council on the mid-north coast, they have stopped burning off at the tip, which makes me realise that my illness has brought about some changes for the better in helping to keep our environment clean. If enough people speak out, changes do occur.

Becoming ill has also helped my family to appreciate their health and to look after it — prevention is better than cure. That is why, in order to stay well, we should all be conscious of exposure to toxic chemicals and why we should eat a good balanced diet of clean, unpolluted food. Our engine is only as good as the clean quality fuel we put into it and the wear, tear and stress we give it. If we treat it gently and well it will last for years.

ME/CFS has changed my way of thinking entirely. I now realise that the things I was so paranoid about were really not important. I have stopped rushing around as I used to do, the house has become a real home not a showplace and I have taken stock of my life, thus sorting out the real priorities. These are life, love, health and giving. I take time out to see the world around me, to appreciate every living creature, to appreciate the beauty of nature and to appreciate my loving family. It is only when we have been very sick that we realise what life really has to offer and no longer take it for granted. We should live each day to the fullest of our capacity whatever that might be.

Making heaps of money does not create instant happiness. It often brings about a great deal of unhappiness. It is the caring and sharing, a bonding together of family and friends and an unselfish attitude that bring true happiness within oneself. The most precious thing you can give to anyone is your time. You cannot buy time, nor can you retrieve it after it is lost. So make the most of it — by helping others you are helping yourself.

Finally, I must emphasise that, no matter what programme

you follow, you *will not get better overnight*. It takes months, sometimes years to regain that lost strength. It took me almost twelve months after exposure to what I suspect was herbicide to regain my strength, and two years after my most serious relapse. Therefore do not become discouraged, take a positive attitude and know that you will eventually overcome most of your problems. Old mother nature has finally found a way to slow me down! I accept that fact. However, I am leading a very fulfilling life, doing a few hours of gardening, walking in the bush in moderation, trout fishing once again, entertaining my family for meals, sewing, minding my granddaughters and writing this book. I make time to relax each day, and have a swim whenever possible. This is indeed a vast improvement from the many, many months I have spent during the last six years being either totally or partially invalided.

Take heart, then — you can do it too!

How we can start to clean up our world

It was not until I began researching ways of rehabilitating myself from my illness that I realised fully the implications of what we are doing to our world. I have always loved natural beauty, and taken for granted the fact that it would always be there to enjoy, now I am not at all sure. It had not occurred to me that I may be living in a hostile environment, we just *presume* that everything we eat, breathe, wear and use is safe. If it is readily obtainable we use it without question. It is now obvious to me that I have been taking far too much for granted. I cannot finish this book without making a plea to everyone to think seriously about our environment — mother earth — which we have taken for granted and abused mercilessly without giving a thought to the consequences of our actions. Our water, land, food and air are already polluted with toxic chemicals owing to our industrialised lifestyle which has changed so rapidly the balances of nature over the past 50 years. All this has taken place in the name of progress. However we are now seeing the effects of the misuse of our world in the 'greenhouse effect' and the depletion of the ozone layer, not to mention the many people being debilitated by diseases such as ME/CFS, asthma, cancer, leukemia, aplastic anaemia, Parkinson's and Alzeheimer's disease, allergies, etc. which are being linked to toxic chemicals.

The unusual weather patterns, the rise in the sea levels, the incidence of skin cancers and the fact that traces of toxic chemicals, including pesticides, have been found as far away as the Antarctic, must make us realise that our continued existence on this planet may become doubtful unless we change our ways. It is going to take an amazing amount of initiative and innovation to change the patterns of our industralised world, by harnessing or inventing others sources of power which are non-pollutant and by changing the 'throw-away consumer society' we have become. Conservation is paramount.

Sewage is a big problem in Sydney. Because of neglect and lack of foresight and planning, our beaches are being rendered unsafe for swimming, our coastal fishing industry is questionable, people are not confident that the fish they purchase or catch is unpolluted and our tourist industry will certainly suffer. Industry has been permitted to dispose of toxic waste via the sewer which has compounded the problem and Sydney sewage has been virtually untreated. How can previous governments have been so negligent? It will cost billions to rectify the situation but we have no choice — it must be done. Full marks to the present New South Wales government for admitting the problem and here's hoping they will follow it through to a safe and efficient conclusion.

Although methods are being created to treat sewage by utilisation of its components as fertilisers etc. and reducing it to clear uncontaminated water, we must play *our* part by respecting the drains and sewers and using them only for the purposes for which they were designed.

The 'wastemaster' was an amazing invention, designed to dispose of our kitchen waste. However this adds to the volume of organic material to be processed as sewage and should be utilised as compost by those of us who have a garden. We rarely use ours today. Toilet and bathroom cleaners also end up in the sewer. Many of these contain toxic chemicals which finish up in the ocean. Just give a little thought as to where it will eventually travel and avoid putting anything down our drains which will pollute our waterways as these are our very source of life.

I watched a neighbour recently cleaning his paint brushes and pots in the gutter. I am sure he did not give a thought to the fact that it would flow down into the creek and damage the wildlife. Even if we bury it in the soil it has to end up somewhere. What a lot of problems our present way of life, although comfortable, has created.

Local councils are acting very irresponsibly by regularly spraying with herbicides to kill grass and weeds. Before the days of herbicides our parks, streets, railway station gardens and ovals were kept magnificently by cutting and mowing instead of killing. Now, chemicals leach into our waterways as soon as it rains and of course end up in our drinking water, our fish, animals and other foods.

Similarly the pest control industry should be encouraged to use only *safe* treatments and we should all insist on this. It is only when the population makes enough noise that governments will be persuaded to insist that chemical companies become more responsible by ceasing to produce toxic products and waste. There are natural safe alternatives.

Do not be persuaded that organochlorines, organophosphates and carbamates are safe. They can have serious effects on humans and cause long-term damage to the environment. Spraying for spider control is a waste of money also. This is in the main ineffective as spiders have pads on their feet which make them immune to any residual surface sprays. A responsible pest controller will tell you that the only way to eradicate spiders is to seek out each nest and treat it individually. However it is mostly unwise to kill spiders as they play a huge part in nature by killing flies and mosquitoes; the spiders in turn provide food for the birds and reptiles and so the cycle of nature continues — when we upset it we pay the penalty. The only way to survive is to work *with* nature. Farmers are realising this and producing crops of grains, fruit and vegetables and raising stock without the use of artificial fertilisers and toxic sprays. They are implementing improved methods of natural farming with great success and less cost. They should be encouraged by us all and so ensure our ultimate survival.

Agricultural spraying of pesticides and artificial fertilisers is causing long-term and far-reaching damage. These pollute the air as well as the land and of course end up in our waterways, oceans, drinking water and our food. They upset the delicate balance of nature and there is abundant evidence of this in the destruction of predator insects, in soil degradation by the destruction of earthworms and bacteria, and in the contamination of our rivers and lakes. Also, artificial fertilisers are causing huge growths of algae thus suffocating all life in many rivers and streams. If only we could all work along with nature before it is too late.

The recent contamination of our export beef is another example of the pesticide residues in our food chain. Toxic drenches, drugs and even hormone treatments are used in the production of our meat and chickens. It seems that *faster and bigger* is considered best. Has anyone considered that flavour and safety might be preferred by the majority of people? Those farmers who are treating their animals with homoeopathy and growing their crops organically are finding that their produce is very much sought after. (I might add that the flavour and sweetness is extremely noticeable.) There is hope for the future but it is really up to us to speak out and demand *clean air*, *clean water* and *clean food*.

I have very dear friends who are farmers. Many years ago when dieldrin was first marketed in this country, one of the family suffered dieldrin poisoning and was extremely ill. He has never used it again and is extremely wary of all such products. He has been raising cattle and sheep and growing wheat very successfully by working along with nature for the thirty years I have known the family, so it can be done, even in these days of mass production.

When we now find that traces of pesticides are to be found in human breast milk we must realise how tenuous the existence of the next generations may be. Many of these chemicals are known to cause cancer, mutations, defects and damage to the nervous and immune systems. Just what are we doing to the human race?

It is most heartening to see celebrities like Meryl Streep taking up this cause in the USA but it is so sad that is has taken so long for us to wake up. We have not quite ruined Australia yet — speak up, don't let it happen, we are fighting for the survival of the next generation.

There is no need to use dangerous chemicals. We managed for generations without them. I have been an avid gardener for many years, having created and landscaped three rather large gardens. I have no need to buy fertilisers nor have I ever needed to use toxic chemicals. Occasionally I use garlic spray on my vegetables. Planting herbs and flowers amongst the vegetables seems to be fairly effective and the occasional chewed leaf doesn't bother me. I am a compost, mulch and leaf-mould extremist. My garden grows too well and I let the bugs, bees and butterflies take their fill. If occasionally something dies , then so be it, it is nature. The lawn clippings are periodically left on the lawn as fertiliser and the leaves are raked off the grass before mowing and put on the garden. Needless to say my garden is a haven for the birds who take their fill with safety. They even drink and splash in my swimming pool which is unchlorinated. The other evening I looked out and saw two large ducks swimming on the pool. It is so important to keep a clean environment to protect every living creature.

Air pollution we can ignore no longer. It is the burning of carbon containing fuels such as wood, coal, gas and oil which produce carbon dioxide. A certain amount of carbon dioxide is necessary for plants to grow because they absorb carbon dioxide and convert it to oxygen. We breathe out carbon dioxide. But according to a scientist at the CSIRO we have reached a worrying level of carbon dioxide in our atmosphere and must cut back the burning of fossil fuels. This applies to us all and to all kinds of burning, including fires, oil heaters, combustion heaters, and gas heaters. These not only produce carbon dioxide, but the last three produce deadly carbon monoxide also.

Carbon monoxide is produced when fossil fuels are burnt with restricted oxygen, i.e. stoves, furnaces, engines, cigarettes, and the worst of all is the motor car. The only way to destroy carbon monoxide is by way of catalytic conversion, which is the process being used in anti-pollution devices on cars and works by burning at a very high temperature.

Fires are necessary for the regeneration of our Australian bush as many seeds are only activated after burning. The Aboriginals, by moving from place to place and by the burning of small sections of bush at a time, kept the balance of nature. We have most certainly upset it.

We have produced an enormous quantity of carbon dioxide and we have removed large sections of forest. It is the young growing trees which absorb the most carbon dioxide. Large-scale planting is obviously required but it is only part of the answer as a large amount of the conversion of carbon dioxide into oxygen occurs via plankton floating on the surface of our oceans. Therefore it is essential that these micro-organisms are not destroyed by pollution (pesticides and herbicides) or by ultraviolet rays.

The recent announcement by the Prime Minister to set

aside millions of dollars over a ten year period to treat soil degradation and to plant thousands of trees is to be applauded. Although many people argued that it was an impossibility to plant such trees in the country due to the need for protection from rabbits and other animals, surely some positive action can be taken. There seem to be too many negative thinkers in this country.

How about BHP and other large manufacturers donating steel stakes and wire mesh to surround these trees? The councils or community service organisations could take charge of the scheme and use the services of unemployed people in country areas for this purpose. It would give them a pride in their country and an involvement in the rebuilding of our environment. This used to be such a positive, innovative and productive country. Perhaps the thought of impending self-destruction may be the catalyst which will bring the country together in a concerted effort to undo the damage we have done. We have the opportunity to lead the world in preserving a safe environment for us all. That does not necessarily mean locking it all away, but it does mean putting back that which we have taken out, by working with what nature provides, and by finding safe methods of agriculture, manufacture and non-pollutant sources of energy.

There are so many things we can do if we take the trouble and really care about the future. Try to persuade those with whom you communicate to see the dangers in continuing our present way of living, *demand* a clean environment both at home and in the workplace and gradually the employers will take notice. The manufacturers will take notice if we boycott their toxic products and the growers will get the message if we insist on pesticide-free food. Governments will legislate to make industry clean up its act if we demand clean *air* and *water*.

Each and every one of us has to start with ourselves — it is not someone else's problem. So take a look in your cupboards — do you really need all those cleaning products? Don't forget, they all flow into our sewers and drains and end up in our waterways and oceans.

Instead of consuming and throwing away, start recycling. Many councils have commenced recycling programmes for glass, plastic drink bottles and paper. It is a marvellous idea and should be extended to many other items as it is in countries overseas, including Holland. There are aluminium and glass depots at many garbage dumps and shopping centres.

Plastics are becoming a big problem both by way of manufacturing processes, toxicity and by way of disposal. I am not convinced that the UV light-sensitive plastic bags are the answer as many will not see the light of day, therefore will not disintegrate. The Smorgon Plastics Recycling in Victoria is recycling plastic. The recycled plastic is marketed as 'Syntal' and is purported to be non-toxic. It is suitable for many situations which previously used wooden slats or logs. Woolworths now have bins outside their stores for plastic waste.

Instead of accepting plastic shopping bags and packaging, take a basket or bag with you. If there is a large quantity of shopping to cope with, place it in the trolley and transfer it to several cardboard cartons kept in the boot of the car. Wrap the garbage which cannot be composted into newspaper and place in your garbage tin.

I keep a carton where I place all the brochures, envelopes, scrap paper, junk mail etc. for recycling. Offices should be encouraged to do this. It is amazing how much waste paper is collected. Supermarkets in the US supply paper carry bags and a minimum of 'cellophane' bags and wraps are being used for packaging overseas. If we used those methods here it would certainly cut down on pollution as we have an enormous amount of waste packaging.

It is no excuse to say that changing our methods of production will cause the loss of jobs. Our changing world has created these problems for years. As one job becomes redundant, another takes its place. We have to learn to cope with change.

This is the challenge of the 21st century. Stand up and be counted. We have the technical resources, we have the innovative spirit, we have a wonderful country filled with natural resources. I hope we have the will to face the challenge.

What you can do

- Stop consuming and throwing away.
- Buy only non-toxic, organic detergents, washing powders, cleaning agents, soaps, shampoos etc, so that we do not pollute our waterways and sewers.
- Demand unbleached paper and recycled paper.
- Demand recycling of all glass and paper products.
- Buy the barest minimum of paper products. Where there is an alternative — such as serviettes, hand-kerchiefs, nappies — buy only cloth which can be laundered.
- Demand products which are non-toxic.
- Demand magazines and books which are not coated with toxic chemicals.
- Demand that industry be innovative and produce only safe products which do not contain toxic chemicals and volatile solvents.
- Stop buying pressure pack products.
- Avoid buying plastic products wherever possible, especially plastic bags.
- Refuse plastic carry bags — take a basket instead.
- Stop using toxic sprays on your gardens and in your homes so that we do not pollute our own environment. We lived successfully without these pollutants for centuries — build on what we have naturally.
- Insist that only natural, safe pest treatments are given by pest controllers.
- Pressure governments to outlaw toxic chemicals.

- Pressure governments to pass laws to force industry to develop ways of production to avoid toxic waste, and to be totally responsible for it.
- Reduce the burning of fossil fuels.
- Encourage the planting of trees until we have created a proper balance of nature.
- Pressure governments to clean up the sewage problems.
- Recycle within your own home as much as possible.
- Buy only what you really *need*.
- Encourage manufacturers to stop unnecessary packaging.
- Walk or ride a bike instead of using the car.
- Encourage industry to be innovative and to look at the production of safe fuels and to invent non-pollutant transport.
- Encourage people to take more responsibility for their own health and to look for more natural, safe remedies. A wholesome diet and lifestyle is the best preventative medicine available.
- Insist that drugs are not handed out willy-nilly when they are known to have severe side effects. Insist that all the side effects be made known to the patient so that he or she can make up their own mind about it.
- Encourage farmers to produce our food without toxic chemicals. *It can be done.*
- Demand clean water, clean air and clean food.
- Encourage people to read the labels and not to use products which contain harmful chemicals.
- Write to governments, councils and manufacturers, insisting that they become absolutely responsible in the production of unpolluted food, non-toxic products, recycling, and that much stricter laws be made regarding toxic waste and air pollution including spraying with pesticides and herbicides.
- Encourage everyone to buy only safe products, to refuse unnecessary packaging, to buy only food wrapped

and packaged in either glass, unbleached paper or 'Cellophane', and to avoid plastic waste to our utmost ability unless it can be guaranteed biodegradable, non-toxic or can be recycled safely.

- Wrap rubbish which cannot be recycled in newspaper and so avoid plastic liners.

- Set an example — speak to your neighbours and friends and join organisations concerned with the environment.

- *Our throw away society must cease* — encourage all Australians to lead the way for the rest of the world.

I   CLINICAL REPORT BY DR ERIC

Therese Whitmore (Trixie) has now been under my care since 1984. She presented then with manifestations of Myalgic Encephalomyelitis/Chronic Fatigue Syndrome. Her symptoms date to June 1983 when she was infected by a virus which is serologically consistent with Influenza B. This led to a diffuse and confusing collection of symptoms including fatigue, aching, tightness and weakness in the trunk muscles, crawling of the skin (formication) and diffuse sweats.

Various strategies were tried from January 1984, including assessment by a neurologist who could find nothing abnormal (although it must be noted that in the previous year, another diagnostic physician had felt there had been viral central nervous system involvement). Blood film was normal.

The following remedies have been given over the five years I have treated her:

Arnica 30 & 200 (Leopard's Bane)
Kali Carbonicum 30 (Carbonate of Potassium)
Bryonia 30 (Wild Hops)
Drosera 30 (Sundew)
Gelsemium 30 (Yellow Jasmine)
Borax 12 (Borate of Sodium)
Chelidonium 30 (Clandine)
Cantharis 30 (Spanish Fly)
Kali Mur 12 (Chloride of Potassium)
Belladonna 30 (Deadly Nightshade)
Acid Sulph 30 (Sulphuric Acid)
Hepar Sulph 30 (Hahnemann's Calcium Sulphide)
Pulsatilla 30 (Wind Flower)
Nux Vomica 30 (Poison-nut)
Echinacea 30 (Purple Cone-flower)
Phytolacca 200 (Poke-root)
Pyrogen 200 (Artificial Sepsin)
Staphylococcia 200 (Staphylococcia)
Lycopodium 30 (Club Moss)
Lachesis 30 (Bushmaster or Surucucu)
Ac Phos 30 (Phosphoric Acid)
Vipera 1m (The German Viper)
Sepia 6, 30, 200 (Cuttle-fish Ink)
Staphysagria 30 (Stavesacre)
Influenza Bac. 30, 1m (Cold & 'Flu Vaccine)
Tuberculinum 30 (A Nosode from Tubercular Abscess)
Arsenicum Alb 30 (Arsenic Trioxide)
Merc Sol 6 (Mercurius)

In view of the antibodies in her blood to Influenza B virus she was given specific homoeopathic immuno-stimulant remedies for Influenza B as well as more general remedies prepared in a series of ascending strengths from her own blood. These gave significant benefit but relapse from overexertion and exposure to toxic chemicals occurred a month later.

Fortunately she did respond quite satisfactorily — at least in the short term — to such standard remedies for muscular weakness as Arnica which has both caused and successfully treated muscular weakness and pain and Kali Carb (Potassium Carbonate) which has an action on intra-cellular potassium flux.

Careful review of her case shows minimal osteoarthritis of the neck as confirmed by X-rays of the neck in 1981. A fairly normal family situation followed her remarriage in 1981.

There is an abundance of evidence in this case of specific maladaptive reaction to environmental chemicals and in particular to pesticides and cigarette smoke. Exposure to these and other noxious chemicals has caused the typical aggravations seen in these cases with days, or even months, of prostrating weakness with muscular pain. These have occurred inadvertently even in the notionally clean environment of her weekender close to the sea, when she inhaled fumes from sprays from neighbouring gardeners as well as pesticide treatments nearby. It is hard to escape the conclusion that these have the force of a 'single blind' clinical experiment. For ethical reasons one would not wish to expose this lady deliberately to chemicals to which she has repeatedly and unpleasantly reacted in the past.

As she is a truthful witness and I have had the benefit of knowing her before and after the attacks and am also familiar with the environment in which she is involved, I have no doubt as to the accuracy of her observations. She has shown a satisfactory response to skilled chiropractic treatment and by maintaining a chemically free environment, with adherence to a diet of food low in pesticide sprays etc., she has regained a substantial measure of her former health. As is typical of these cases, this has occurred over a five year cycle whereby the patient appears outwardly to be normal, but still is quite prone to relapse on exposure to chemicals to which he or she has become intolerant.

Following discussion with leaders in this field, it is my belief that patients with this condition, often of a driving and highly self-motivating temperament, sustain a viral infection which alters the balance between helper and suppressor cells in the blood. Exposure to certain chemicals at this time, such as pesticides or formaldehyde from, for example, self-carboning paper or tobacco smoke, may lead to a sensitisation which is not directly mediated through the IgE pathway. Thus, it is not possible to determine these chemical intolerances by the standard scratch tests. However provocation testing is inevitably positive but of course leads to an intense aggravation of the patient's symptoms. I no longer perform these tests for ethical reasons.

Following productive discussions with Trixie we prepared a question-

naire, the results of which will be included in this book. The symptoms
gathered are remarkably similar to those obtained by wider surveys
performed by the Departments of Immunology at certain Sydney teaching
hospitals and in smaller surveys performed by clinicians of my acquaintance
in the UK.

Trixie Whitmore manifests many of the symptoms of ME/CFS and has
followed the clinical course typical of this illness. It is a sad fact of life that
many chronic illnesses follow a standard pattern, that is, in five years time,
one third are cured, a third are the same and one third are worse. I believe
this ratio holds as good for ME/CFS as it does for diabetes and rheumatoid
arthritis. Ultimately the patient's own attitude towards their illness and the
lessons learned lead to the changes necessary to effect a cure.

All the skilled chiropractic, homoeopathy and nutrition may merely
assist in this process of inner healing, but are not responsible in themselves
for the ultimate healing, which in my personal opinion stems from that
great well of healing within us, that some of us wish to call God.

Questionnaire for ME/CFS Sufferers

This Questionnaire is for Myalgic Encephalomyelitis sufferers who would
like to participate in a survey to see if there is any possibility that the disease
is linked with 20th century lifestyle or chemicals. (The answers, expressed
as percentages, are in bold.)

Did you have a severe virus before showing ME symptoms? **60% Yes**
Please state what type of virus, e.g. glandular fever, hepatitis, influenza, etc.
All three were mentioned, plus Ross River Fever
Did you take antibiotics during or just after this virus? **65% Yes**
Please state which one. **Broad spectrum antibiotics**
Did you take, or were you taking, any other drugs during or just prior to
this illness?
Please state which one(s). **5% variable**
Were you taking any steroids, e.g. cortisone? **3%**
Please state which one. **cortisone**
Do you take the contraceptive pill, or were you taking it at the time? **20%**
Have you had any innoculations, or vaccinations either for overseas travel,
or against diseases (e.g. flu) just before becoming ill?
If so please state which one(s). **10% variable including tick anti-toxin**
Was your house, garden (or neighbour's) or place of work sprayed with
pesticide a short time before becoming ill? If so, which pesticide, and how
long before your illness? **70% variable including aerial spray, pesticides
and herbicides**
Had you been exposed to Baygon, surface sprays, garden sprays,
napthalene, paint, Dettol, disinfectant, bleach or any other strong-smelling

chemical you can remember prior to becoming ill? (this could include a large dose of cigarette smoke). **80% variable**

If so, which one(s) and for how many days/weeks/months. **Napthalene, disinfectant, Baygon, dichlorvos, chlorpyrifos, kerosene, phenol, gas, aerial sprays, Round Up, tear gas, cigarettes, and, tested insecticides at work.**

Do any smells or fumes particularly worry you or make you agitated? **Except for one, all said Yes**

If so please tick the chemicals below and indicate to what degree (mild, intense or overwhelming) they affected you.

Phenol	65% intense
Napthalene	68% intense
Cigarette smoke	95% intense
Flyspray	90% intense
Baygon	90% intense
Detergents	60% intense
Petrol	90% intense
Kerosene	75% intense
Moulds	55% intense
Paints	75% intense
Glues	70% intense
Gas	60% intense
Diesel	80% intense
Garden spray	85% intense
Pesticide spray	95% intense
Hair spray	70% intense
Shampoo	40% intense
Pressure packs	80% intense
Cosmetics	55% intense
Deodorant	60% intense
Perfumes	85% intense
Cleaning fluids	75% intense
Bleach	65% intense
Chlorine	70% intense
Dettol	85% intense
Plastic	65% intense
Vinyl	40% intense
Synthetic fabrics	50% intense
New carpet	75% intense
Newspapers	45% intense
Magazines	55% intense
Books	20% intense
Polishes	75% intense

Any other (please state) **felt pens, Scotchguard, wood stains, methylated spirits, photocopiers, formaldehyde, air conditioners, department stores, 'dope', liquid paper, septic effluent**

Did you notice any smells or fumes bothering you before you either contracted a severe virus or ME? **97% no, 2% yes, 1% unknown**
Did you notice any smells or fumes bothering you after you contracted a severe virus or ME? **98% yes**
Have you experienced a sore, dry nose and/or throat after inhaling fumes which bothered you? **70% yes**
Were you very thirsty after such inhalation? **90% yes**
Did you experience any burning or crawling sensation just under the skin, particularly on the arms or legs? **70% yes**
Did your eyes water, especially at night, after such exposure? **50% yes**
Did you get a severe headache after such exposure? **60% yes**
Did you or do you have candida or thrush? If so, was it of the genitals, mouth or rectum? Please indicate which one. **75% yes, variable**
Did ME come on suddenly or gradually? **60% suddenly, 30% gradually**
Do you suffer from constipation or loose bowel movements? **65% yes**
Do you have indigestion or bloating? **90% yes**
Are you aware that you have any food allergies? **80% yes**
If so please state which ones. **Many and varied including yeast, MSG, moulds**
Does any other member of your family have ME? **25% yes**
Were you under a great amount of stress at the time you contracted ME? **50% yes**
Does your family accept the fact that you have a serious illness and support and assist you? **65% yes**

Thank you for completing this questionnaire.
All information will be treated in strictest confidence.

Author's note

Please note that although people did tick products/smells which worried them, not everyone gave the degree of aggravation therefore I have recorded them under *intense* as being an average. However, quite a large percentage had *overwhelming* aggravation to Baygon, petrol, kerosene, pesticide and cigarette smoke.

Also some of the participants neglected to fill in some of the questions and one person stated that she had not used any of the products mentioned for years. I would presume that she had a good reason for this, however I could not include her in the affirmatives, but had to include her in the negatives.

Therefore the percentages noted in the questionnaire are approximate and cannot be absolutely accurate.

III Directory of organisations and product sources

I have compiled this list, with much help, from my own contacts. It was correct at the time of going to press. However, you will almost certainly find other sources.

Alternative therapies, medicines and ointments

Homoeopathic doctors
To find a homoeopathic doctor in your area
(02) 686 2554

This telephone number will put you in touch with a medical practitioner who practices homoeopathy, and covers the whole of Australia and New Zealand. Unfortunately there is a scarcity of these practitioners in the country areas.

Martin and Pleasance
137 Swan Street
Richmond 3121
PO Box 2054
(03) 427 7422

For homoeopathic medicines and books, ask at your health food store.

Think Twice
37 Hill Street
Roseville NSW 2069
(02) 416 7997

Herb of Life
Eungai Rail
NSW 2441
(065) 69 0837

Nature Spirit Herbal
    Products Pty Ltd
PO Box 85
Byron Bay NSW
(066) 84 7326

Newton's Pharmacy
119 York Street
Sydney NSW
(02) 267 7889, 264 1653

*Herbal preparations
Mail orders by phone
    Australia-wide*

Smoker's Clinic
St Vincent's Hospital
Darlinghurst NSW 2010
(02) 339 1111

For other help to give up smoking, contact the Quit for Life Programme in your state, or the Department of Health.

ME/CFS Societies

ME/CFS Society of NSW Inc.
PO Box 645,
Mona Vale 2103
(02) 439 6026

ME/CFS Society, Inc.
   South Australia
GPO Box 383
Adelaide 5001
(08) 49 1913

M.E. Syndrome Society,
   Queensland
PO Box 12,
Oxenford 4210
(07) 341 6190

M.E.C.F. (ID)S.
   Society of WA
PO Box 240
Greenwood 6024
(09) 483 6667

ME/CFS Society Victoria
PO Box 7,
Moonee Ponds 3039
(03) 852 0054

ME Society ACT
Community Centre, Wisdom St,
Hughes 2605
(062) 81 2983

Western Australia
Mr Peter Brown, (09) 342 3179
Urgent Pager 483 6667
(affiliated with ME/CFS
   Society of NSW Inc)

Tasmania
Please contact ME/CFS
   Society Victoria

Blood Tests

Doctors who will arrange chemical blood analysis through ToxIx chemical analysis
3/488 The Entrance Rd.,
Erina Heights 2260
(043) 65 1063 Fax (043) 67 6099
At present blood is sent to USA. Efforts are presently under way to provide the same service in Australia, hopefully by January 1990. This should reduce the cost substantially.

NEW SOUTH WALES

The Special Environment
   Allergy Clinic,
Manly Waters
   Private Hospital,
17 Cove Ave,
Manly 2095
Dr Mark Donohue
Dr John Marshall
Dr Joachim Fluhrer
(02) 977 5577

Complimentary Medicine
   Association
41 Boundary Street,
Rushcutters Bay 2011
(02) 357 5474

Macquarie Pathology will collect blood in NSW and Queensland

QUEENSLAND

Dr Barry Ryan
622 Lutwyche Rd,
Brisbane 4000
(07) 357 6744

Dr David Spall
Suite 59, Silverton Place,
101 Wickham Terrace,
Brisbane 4000
(07) 831 2277

Dr Kevin Treacy
Suite 2A Evandale
   Medical Chambers,
45 Bundall Rd,
Surfers Paradise 4217
(075) 38 2288

VICTORIA

Dr Colin Little
324 Stephenson Road
Mt Waverley Vic. 3149
(03) 888 1345

Dr Robert Allen
Suite 5, 90 Mitcham Rd,
Donvale 3111
(03) 842 8611

Dr Michael Glasby
221 Wonga Rd,
Warranwood 3134
(03) 876 3930

SOUTH AUSTRALIA
Dr Margaret Taylor
4 Baliol Street,
College Park 5069
(08) 363 1557

WESTERN AUSTRALIA
Dr William Barnes
174 Hampton Road,
South Fremantle 6162
(09) 33 6221

Information Regarding Toxic Chemicals

The Total Environment Centre
18 Argyle Street
Sydney NSW 2000
(02) 27 8476

*This centre has a library of information and will give advice regarding
dangerous chemicals.*
*'The A to Z of Chemicals' is available from them and is very informative
although I would not recommend using kerosene as suggested.*

Pest Controllers

Systems Pest Management Pty Ltd
PO Box 110
Leichhardt NSW 2040
564 1614
and
29 Hughes Ave
Lawson NSW 2783
(047) 592 498
and
PO Box 123
Palmyra WA 6157
(09) 339 5760

Any queries regarding pest treatments should be directed to this firm
who will advise as to safe treatments. They have worked in conjunction
with the Total Environment Centre who will also advise.

Interior decorating

DLW Flooring (Linoleum)
Their distributors are:
  Greig Bros Pty Ltd
  Sydney (02) 647 2955
  Melbourne (03) 429 1044
  Adelaide (08) 297 8311
  Brisbane (07) 345 7800
  Perth (09) 446 8100

Bio-Products Australia Pty Ltd
  25 Aldgate Terrace
  Bridgewater SA 5155
  (08) 339 1923

Aglaia and Livos Paints
  Ecological Building and Living
  124 Station Street
  Blackheath 2785
  (047) 87 7554

The Clean House Effect
  345 King Street
  Newtown 2042
  (02) 516 4681

Their distributors in other states are as follows:

New South Wales
Lionell O'Neill
  Helios Enterprises P/L
  65 Derwent St
  Glebe 2037
  (02) 660 2555

Mr Alexander Taylor
  Shop 3, 13 Kalinda Rd
  Bullaburry 2784
  Work (047) 591 355
  Home (047) 571 940

Mrs Kathryn Simpson
  207 Boundary Rd
  Oakville 2765
  Home (045) 736 032
  Work (02) 644 1233

Alexander Schubert
  Tuckpointing Masonry
  Maintenance
  10 Egmont Rd
  Medlow Bath 2780
  (047) 881 117

Mr Graham von Laue
  C. & G. Insulations
  Lot 38, Melville St
  Culcairn 2660
  (060) 298 529

Debo. Guilbner
  PO Box 278
  Moruya 2537
  (044) 743 736

Victoria
Steven Engroville
  Going Solar
  320 Victoria St
  Melbourne 3051
  (03) 328 4123

Mr & Mrs Roth
  Allergy Aid Centre
  325 Chapel St
  Prahran 3181
  (03) 529 7348

Mrs Margaret Webster
  Naturally Aware
      (Hills Health Products)
  (Waldorf School)
  133 Union Rd
  Surrey Hills 3127
  (03) 898 3591

Mr Tony Fiorenza
  1 Sightfoot St
  Shepparton 3630
  (058) 311 698

South Australia

Rodney Twiss
  109 Glen Osmond Rd
  Eastwood 5063
  (08) 272 1981

Dawn Futons — Brett Craig
  72 Bacon St
  Hindmarsh 5007
  (08) 464 598

All in good Mine
      — Linda and Paul
  35 Wheatland St
  Seacliff 5049
  (08) 296 5876

Kim Atkinson
  Natural Technology Systems
  120 Prospect Rd
  Prospect 5082
  (08) 344 7298

Queensland

Rod and Wendy Butler
  BIO Distributors Qld.
  PO Box 86
  Samford 4520
  (07) 289 1663

Western Australia

Mr Ray Tauss
  16 Crowea St
  Greenwood 6024
  (09) 447 9053

Mr John McBain
  PO Witchliffe 6286
  (097) 572 460

Cleaning products, toiletries and cosmetics

Brot Bodyline
  PO Box 321
  Moruya NSW 2537
  (144) 738 782

Caring Products
  446 Victoria St,
  North Melbourne, Vic. 3051
  (03) 749 4673

Helios Enterprises Limited
  65 Derwent Street
  Glebe NSW 2937
  (02) 660 2555

Herbonics Australia
  29 Stewart Street
  Richmond South Vic 3121
  (03) 429 3733

Naural Oil Workers Co-Op
   PO Box 125
   St Peters NSW 2044

Simple Products
   Smith and Nephew
   (Australia) Pty Ltd
   211 Wellington Rd
   Clayton Vic 3162
   (03) 566 1200

Weleda
   2D Elizabeth Bay
      Gardens
   Elizabeth Bay
   NSW 2011
   (02) 357 1554

Women's Health Advisory Service
   187 Glenmore Road
   Mail Order service
   (PO Box 217)
   Paddington NSW 2021
   (02) 331 5014

Natural Product Distributors
   113 Frederick Street
   Welland SA 5007
   (08) 340 0288

Sunotex Pty Ltd
   PO Box 919
   Clarence St
   Sydney 2000
   (02) 267 7775

Whole Harvest
   8 Point Street
   PO Box 180
   Pyrmont 2009
   (02) 552 1595

Melrose Laboratories
   3/24 Lexton Road
   Box Hill 3128
   (03) 898 9571

Beverages

Botobolar Vineyard Pty Ltd
   PO Box 212
   Mudgee NSW 2850
   (063) 73 3840

The Colonial Beverage Company
   Batar Creek Road
   Kendall NSW 2439
   (Norfolk Punch)
   (065) 59 4464

Mount Vincent Mead
   'Kinlochleven'
   (PO Box 170)
   Mudgee 2850
   (063) 72 3184

Madura Tea
   Madura Tea Estates Pty Ltd
   Clothiers Creek
   Condong NSW 2484
   (066) 77 7310

Baking Powder (low allergy)

Cabinlee Kitchen
310 Main South Road
Croydon Park 5008
(08) 46 3228

'Cellophane' bags

Write to:
Trixie Whitmore
PO Box 266
Pymble NSW 2073

Organic Produce Available in Australia

I have been assisted by various people in the preparation of this list of suppliers of organic foods and particularly by the Natural Health Society of Australia (Tel: (047) 215068) who have allowed me to re-print the information contained in Volume 2 No. 1 Dec/Jan 1988/89 of their magazine *Natural Health*, for which I sincerely thank the Editor.
The produce from each outlet below will, in most cases, be fruit and vegetables, grains, nuts, seeds, cheeses and fruit juices.

AUSTRALIA WIDE
Biodynamic rice and other grains, nuts seeds, cheeses and fruit juices.
By mail order from:
Biodynamic Marketing Co. Ltd.
Main Road, Powelltown, Vic. 3797

Helios Enterprises P/L (Demeter)
65 Derwent St. Glebe 2937 (02) 660 2555

SYDNEY
Home Delivery
The Organic Delivery,
    Western Suburbs. 221 7528
Mary's Organics 958 3947
More Health 764 2805
Simon Langoulant 365 0463
Richard Jacobsen 977 0458

Restaurants

Annandale
    Lurlene's Cafe,
    85 Booth Street,
    660 0203

Glebe
    Iku,
    25a Glebe Point Road
    692 8720

The Rocks
Rockpool Restaurant,
109 George St
252 1888

Retailers

Balmain
Helmuts Health Food Barn
312 Darling Street
810 4015

Balmain Markets — Organic farm produce each Saturday.

Bondi Junction
Macro Whole Foods,
328 Oxford Street
Bondi Junction
389 7611

Caringbah
Simply Organic,
67 Parthenia Street
524 0608

Chatswood
Russells Natural Food Markets
234 Victoria Ave
411 1779

Spring Street Fruit Market
15 Spring Street
419 6024

Clovelly
Foods Naturale
29 Burnie Street
664 1900

Cremorne
The Good Health Shop
880 Military Road
969 9131

Quality Meat Shop
47a Spofforth Street
909 3383
Bio-dynamic beef, lamb, pork
chickens etc.

Cronulla
Cronulla Health Foods
Mareeba Arcade, 35 Cronulla St.
523 2488

Crows Nest
Annabelles Natural Food Store
18 Willoughby Road
906 6377

Dee Why
Russells Health Foods
11 Oaks Road
982 4442

Double Bay
Raw Energy
19 Cross Street
32 4399

Cosmopolitan Fruit Market
22 Knox Street
327 6068

Dural
Warrah Farm
20 Harris Road
651 2411

Edgecliff
Harris Farm Market
Eastpoint Food Fair
328 7782

Engadine
Whey of Life
69 Station Street
520 3169

Flemington
Flemington Markets B Block
764 3988

Harris Farm Markets
Flemington Markets G Shed
764 2966

Glebe
Russells Natural Food Markets
55 Glebe Point Road
660 8144

Demeter Bakery
65 Derwent Street
660 2555
Bio-dynamic grain, gluten free
bread, fruit & juices

Jannali
Jannali Health Foods
566 Box Road
528 9759

Lilyfield
Steve Alexander
68–72 Cecily Street
958 3322, 810 3164
Organic fruit & vegetable
wholesaler

Liverpool
PJ's Health Foods
Shop 12, Liverpool Plaza,
Macquarie Street
821 1191

Londonderry
Shalom Cottage
52 Trahlee Road
(045) 78 4196

Miranda
Parkside Fruit Market
525 3416

Mona Vale
The Good Health Shop
7 Waratah St.,
997 7513

Mosman
The Good Health Shop,
880 Military Road,
969 9131

Harris Farm Market
70A Vista Street
960 3548

Neutral Bay
Neutral Bay Fruitland
Cnr. Grosvenor & Young Sts
909 1199

Newport
Sirius Natural Foods Store
313b Barrenjoey Road
997 4262

Newtown
Newtown Markets
Saturdays only

Macro Wholefoods
170 King Street
550 5668

North Avalon
Searl's Health Foods
27 Albert Road
918 2803

Northbridge
Wholehearted
Shop 5 Northbridge Plaza
958 6539

Paddington
Paddington Markets
Organic farm produce each
Saturday

Pennant Hills West
West Pennant Hills Health Foods
14 Castle Hill Road
84 4113

Pymble
CHEM-FREE Meats
1094 Pacific Highway
44 2199
*Meat, chicken, fruit, vegetables,
jams, juices, grains, sauces.*

Randwick
Health & Healing
22 Perouse Road
399 3538
Alex Slow Foods (Bakery)
399 3538
*Organically produced bread &
grain products*

Redfern
Paddy's Markets
365 0463

Rockdale
Russells Health Foods,
463 Princes Highway
59 1011

Rouse Hill
Tebutts Open Range Eggs
90 Schofields Road
629 1139
*Open range chickens, chicken &
duck eggs. At Christmas, open-
range turkeys. Cannot guarantee
that all grain feed in organic, farm
is organic.*

Warriewood
Warriewood Fruit Market
Shop 35 Warriewood Shopping
Centre
913 7386

Wentworthville
Big Apple Fruit Market
48 Dunmore Street
631 3858

Willoughby
Harris Farm Markets
201 High Street
958 5520

Co-operatives
Chris Sheard
606 5960

Debbie Callaghan
158 Pittwater Road
MANLY 977 4304

Fruit Co-Op
19 Palace Street
PETERSHAM 569 7753

John Hunter
660 1122

Marie Indja
9 Bedford Crescent
COLLAROY 971 0309

NEW SOUTH WALES

Home Delivery
WARILLA
Paul & Vicky Miller
10 Raymond Ave
(042) 964 150

Retailers
Armidale
Harvest Wholefoods
(067) 721 869

Bowral
Scoopful of Good Health
4 Boolwey St
(048) 613 913

Byron Bay
Michael Reid
Epicentre Shopping Complex
(066) 876 048

Santos Trading
Lawson Street
(066) 857 071

Coffs Harbour
High Street Fruit Barn
124 High Street
(066) 523 543

Cooma
The Organic Garden
95 Commissioner Street
(064) 524 974

Glossodia
Bountiful Harvest
Spinks Road
(045) 79 6778

Katoomba
Mals Quality Fruit
Shop 2, 48 Park Street
(047) 82 1210

Kyogle
Kyogle Organic Growers
272 Summerland Way
(066) 322 244

Laurieton
Camden Haven Fruit
& Vegetable Market
Shop 4/64 Bold Street
(065) 59 8296

Leura
Leura Village Store
157 The Mall
(047) 84 1438

Lismore
Fundamental Foods
104 Keen Street,
(066) 216 760

Macksville
Sunflowers Natural Food
6B Cooper Street
(065) 681 262

Moruya
Moruya Fruit & Vegetable Market
11 Church Street
(044) 742 451

Mullumbimby
Santos Trading
89 Stuart Street
(066) 842 410

Murwillumbah
Santos Trading
Main Street
(066) 722 715

Pambula
Organically Yours
26A Quondola Street
(064) 957 085

Narooma
Naturebound
Lynch's Arcade
(044) 76 1130

Newcastle
Natural Tucker
Darby Street, Cooks Hill
(049) 29 1229

Hamilton Fruit Barn
135A Beaumont Street, Hamilton
(049) 615 455

Saratoga
Saratoga Fruit Market
Shop 5 Saratoga Shopping Village
(043) 691 059

Springwood
Natural Food Supplies
127 Macquarie Road
(047) 511 842

Taree
Paul Turner
Rear of Rumours Coffee Lounge
(065) 532581

Wagga
Budget Wholefoods
Shop 8 & 9 Neslo Arcade
(069) 22 7394

Co-Operatives
Karen Medbury
(062) 950 832

Bathurst
Susan Herald
15 Morriset Street
(063) 316 154

Condobolin
Mark Spears,
Jones Road
(068) 95 3834

Wentworth Falls
For Food and Thought
The Centre, Station St
(047) 57 3222

Tree of Life
(047) 57 3222

Wingham
Wingham Natureland
Shop 12, Stones Corner Complex
(065) 570 211

Wollongong
Back to Basics,
383 Princes Highway, Woonona
(042) 835 352

All Organic
77 Purr Purr Ave, Warilla
(042) 962 676

Wyoming
Wyoming Fruit Market,
464 Pacific Highway,
(043) 284 551

Wyong
Central Coast Organics
Shop 14, Railway Square
(043) 512 378

ACT
Canberra
ACT Organic Canberra
   Home Delivery
(062) 47 8892
ANU Nutrition Society,
ANU Campus,
Kingsley Street
(062) 57 1186

MELBOURNE
Blackburn
Angelo's Organic &
   Bio Natureland,
92 South Pde
677 3030

Caulfield
Fruiterama,
57A Kooyong Road
(H) 534 6400,
(B) 500 9685

Caulfield South
Produce Plus,
241 Bambra Road
523 5647

Cheltenham
The Wade Family
   Distributors,
364 Reserve Road
583 4493

Clifton Hill
Vic Market Organics,
11 Hilton Street
482 2052

Collingwood
Organic Fruit &
   Vegetable Co-op
419 9926

Croydon North
Peter Thurlows Biodynamic
& Organic Produce,
McAdam Square 53 761

ACT Organic
Unit 12/25 Darling Street
Mitchell (062) 418 290

Joseph Alias
Shop 12, Fishwick Market
(062) 958 938

Croydon South
Eastfield Health Foods,
39 The Mall 723 0257

Elwood
Elwood Fruit Bowl,
24 Ormond Road
531 6305.
Natural Health Supplies,
78 Ormond Road
531 7577

Ferntree Gully
Gully Greengrocer,
101 Station Street
758 8650

Fitzroy
Organic Fruit & Vegetable
   Co-Op,
222 Brunswick Street
419 9926

Footscray
Organic Wholesalers,
Footscray Markets

Glen Waverly
The Organic Shop,
102 Kingsway
561 8030

Hampton
Chris's Fruit Land,
373 Hampton Street
597 0392

Hawthorn
Mediterranean Fruit
    Supply,
42 Church Street
861 6570

Hurstbridge
Hurstbridge Organic
    Fruit Shop,
Shop 6
Main Road
718 2174

Montrose
Montrose Fruit &
    Health,
914 Mt Dandenong
Tourist Road
728 1377

Mt Evelyn
Advance Fruit &
    Health Supplies,
4 York Road
736 3142

Noble Park
Tony & Tina's
Org. & Bio. Fruit & Veg,
2 Buckley Street
546 1027

Pascoe Vale
Natural Health Supplies,
23 Springhall Pde
386 0749

Prahran
Ceres Wholefoods,
116 Chapel Street
529 206
Greens & Grains
Health Foods,
123 Grenville Street
514 256

Richmond
Organic Grocery,
310 Bridge Road. 429 9219

Ringwood
Healthy Life Ringwood,
5 Civic Place
870 2010
Ringwood Gourmet,
Shop 23,
New Ringwood Market
879 5072

Ripponlea
Ripponlea Health
    Foodstore,
77 Glen Eira Road
523 6416

Surrey Hills
Food Sensitivity Shop,
137 Union Road
890 1292

Upwey
Upwey Health Foods,
4/9-21 Main Street
754 4581

Warrandyte
Home Grown Organic
    Produce,
Shop 3,
90 Melbourne Hill Rd
844 1126

Werribee
Produce Plus,
Shop 8,
Hoppers Crossing

VICTORIA — COUNTRY

Ballarat
Barbara's Organics,
9 Rippon Street,
Ballarat North
(053) 323 344

Bendigo
Bendigo Health Foods,
74 Mitchell Street
(054) 431 910

Cockatoo
Cockatoo Vegie patch,
Shop 2-4 Bailey Road
Home (059) 688 350,
B (059) 688 426

Geelong
Wholefoods Co-Operative,
2 McLarty Place
(052) 215 421

Healesville
Bellbird Organic Fruit
& Vegetables,
181 Maroondah Hwy
(059) 624 081

Lorne
Lorne Greens Fruit &
Vegetables,
Mountjoy Pde
Home (052) 891 531,
B (052) 891 383

Mornington
Don't Panic It's Organic,
3 Blake Street
(059) 756 999

Timboon
Timboon Farmhouse
Cheese,
Ford & Fells Road
All types of bio-dynamic cheeses

BRISBANE

Wholesaler
Sunstate Organic
Wholesalers,
M.S. 2078,
Palmwoods
(071) 459 442

Brisbane
Robert Hennig,
Eldar Trading
892 2922

Breakfast Creek Wharf
Sundays organic market

Cleveland
Here's Health,
Shop 10 Middle Street,
Woolies Complex
286 4219

Eagle Junction
Eagle Junction Health
Foods,
Junction Road
357 6892

Kyogle Organic Growers,
Brisbane Shop,
(07) 870 4733

Red Hill
Good Foods Co-Op,
78 Arthur Terrace
369 0898

Springwood
The Health Connection,
Arndale Shopping Centre,
Cinderella Drive
209 3864

Toowong
Toowong Wholefoods,
Cnr. Haig & Bangalla Streets
371 7585

West End
Better Health Foods,
143 Boundary Road
844 7961

QUEENSLAND — COUNTRY

Boonah
Healthy's Wholefoods
& Remedies,
8A Railway Street
(075) 632 991

Buderim
Buderim Health Foods,
39 Main Street
(071) 452 625

Eumundi
Eumundi Health Foods,
Main Street,
Eumundi
(071) 428 666

Gympie
Gympie Health Foods,
Shop 140 Mary Street
(071) 822 913
Gympie Organic Market,
No. 24 Nash Street
(071) 826 223

W'Gabba
Prevention Health
Foods,
39 Logan Road
393 0534

Wynnum
Lyndon Fruit Shop,
273 Sibley Road,
Wynnum West
396 1093

Killarney
Killarney Health Foods,
Pine Street
(076) 641 435

Maleny
Maple Street Co-Op Ltd.,
Maple Street
(071) 942 088

Mapleton
Black-All Range Co-Op,
Obi Obi Road
(071) 457 397

Miami
Raphael Pure Foods,
Cnr Hillcrest & Kallay St
(075) 525 644

Nambour

Basics Co-Op. Soc. Ltd.,
Porters Lane
(071) 414 112
Nambour Health Foods,
29B Howard Street
(071) 412 006

Noosa Junction

Noosa Health Foods,
Emerald House,
Sunshine Beach Rd
(071) 473 053

Stanthorpe

Heather's Health Shop
(076) 811 575

Toowoomba

Good Farmer John's
(076) 382 958

Townsville

Parkside Gardens Fruit
 Shop,
Parkside Gardens
Shopping Centre,
19 Fraser Avenue,
Cranbrook
(077) 737 255

Warwick

Billywacs Health Foods,
44 Perry Street
Home (076) 661 688

ADELAIDE

Adelaide

Adelaide Central Market,
Stall 62 and others
Clearlight Wholefoods,
201 Rundle Street
223 6362

Basket Range

Tim Marshall
390 341
*Grower prepared to grow for
families*

Brompton

The Hindmarsh City Farm
461 884
*Grower prepared to grow for
families*

Maylands

From the Earth,
195 Magill Road
363 1911

Norwood

Zuccini Brothers Fruiterers,
144B Magill Road
362 7786

Parkside

Unley Health Foods
271 1595

Stirling

The Organic Market,
Shop 5, 5 Druids Ave
339 4835

SOUTH AUSTRALIA — COUNTRY

Mt Barker

Four Seasons,
Gawler Street

Two Wells
Peter Thompson
(085) 202 412
*Grower prepared to grow for
families*

PERTH

Kelmscott
Fruit Loop,
100 Brookton Highway
390 7026
*Grow own organic produce
and will deliver as far north
as Yanchep and as far south
as Rockingham*

Sawyers Valley
New Hope Organic Farm,
Clint Woodward
295 2126
*Fruit and pecans grown and
delivered to co-ops and families in the Perth area*

WESTERN AUSTRALIA

No list is available. There
are a few local outlets
selling organic
produce at health food
shops and fruit and
vegetable outlets.

HOBART

Cygnet
Mimosa Wholefoods,
Mary Street
95 1931

Geeveston
Sunflower Wholefood
and Coffee Shop,
Church Street
97 1767

Wembley
Organic Growers Assoc,
239 Jersey Street
387 1269, 451 4282

Glenorchy
Healthy Life Health
   Food Store,
48 Grove Road
72 4665

Hobart
Healthy Life Health
   Food Store,
206 Centrepoint
34 9167

Prasad Wholefoods,
249 Sandy Bay Road
23 7540

Kingston
Yum Yum Tree Health
    Shop & Solariums,
23 Beach Road
29 5253

TASMANIA — COUNTRY

Deloraine
The Healthwise Shoppe,
86 Emu Bay Road
(003) 62 2515

Launceston
Healthway Food Co.,
134 York Street
(003) 31 7779
UWU Wholefoods,
Cnr Frederick and
Wellington Streets

West Hobart
Eumarrah Cafe,
39 Barrack Street

Ulverstone
Leven River Traders,
37 King Edward Street
(004) 25 4884

Each of the following should be able to give information regarding organic produce and its availability.

Victoria
Organic Retailers and
Growers Association of
Victoria
(03) 737 9565

Western Australia
Fruit Loop in Perth grow
and deliver organic produce
(09) 390 7026

Queensland
Brisbane Organic
Growers' Inc.
PO Box 236, Lutwyche 4030
The Good Foods Co op
(07) 369 0898

South Australia
The Zucchini Brothers
(08) 362 7786

Whilst visiting Laurieton New South Wales health food store I was introduced to an agricultural newspaper being produced by the organic farmers of the country, *ECO-AG The Future for Farming*. Information regarding this newspaper can be obtained from Eco-Ag, PO Box 552, Fortitude Valley, 4006, Queensland.

Also farmers, scientists, researchers and representatives of federal and state governments presented a timely and vital overview of the economics, market potential and certification requirements for organic food systems at a conference, ECO-AG 89.

A bound volume of all papers presented at ECO-AG 89 is available at $18.00 per copy from the above address. Cheque made payable to ECO-AG 89.

Other Products

Bedding — non-allergenic
Allersearch

New South Wales
8 Marco Ave
Revesby NSW 2212
(02) 771 6944

Victoria
2/194 Whitehorse Rd
Blackburn VIC
(03) 894 1888

Electro magnetic clips
Tony Narracott
Sun Medical Equipment
 Centre
224 Victoria Rd
Rozelle NSW 2030
(02) 818 1533

Recycling
Smorgon Plastics Recycling
413 Somerville Road
West Footscray Vic 3012
(03) 316 5227

Swimming pool purifier
Aquamatics Pty Ltd
PO Box 54
Seaforth NSW 2092

Water purifiers
Cartier Water Purifiers
20 Crystal St
Rozelle NSW 2039
(02) 818 5576

Allergy Aid Centre
325 Chapel St
Prahran 3181
(03) 529 7348

Quick shopping list of environmentally safe products

Health Food Stores

Herbon Dishwashing Detergent
Herbon Dishwasher Powder
Herbon Laundry Powder or
    Liquid
Pre-wash Stain Remover
Multi-Purpose Cleaner (trigger
    bottle)
Herbon Shampoo — Ginseng
Herbon Conditioner
Herbon Personal and/or Herbon
    Baby Soap
Herbon Deodorant or The
    Natural Alternative Herbal
    Deodorant
Weleda shampoos, conditioner,
    baby talc, cream and lotion,
    massage oil, shaving cream
    and lotion and toothpaste
Golden Wattle Shampoo
Golden Wattle Conditioner
Blackmores Herbal Toothpaste
Brot Bodyline soap and shampoo
Bugg-Off Insect Spray &
    Repellent
Tea tree oil
Lavender oil
Natural honey
Tahini (organically grown)
Soy sauce (including wheat free)
    packed in glass
Olive oil, apricot oil, wheat germ
    oil, avocado oil (packed in
    glass)
Unbleached toilet rolls
Organically grown stoneground
    flour
Low allergy baking powder
    (aluminium free)
Naturally dried fruits
    (unsulphured)
Nuts
Organically-grown brown rice
Organically-grown rolled oats

Herbal teas
Rock salt
Dried Herbs
Natural live culture yoghurt
Bread baked with organically
    grown flour
Fruit juices organically grown
    (packed in glass)
Free-range eggs
Free-range chickens
Norfolk Punch
Seeds for sprouting
Cider Vinegar
Cornflour
Freshly ground peanut butter
Organically grown fruit and
    vegetables (see list in book)
Organically grown meat (see list)
Bio-dynamic butter and cheese
    (when available)
And remember to keep asking
    for organically-grown produce!

Supermarket

Aware Laundry Powder
Sunlight/Velvet Laundry Soap
Sunlight/Velvet Laundry Powder
Bi-carb of soda
Unbleached toilet paper
Greaseproof paper (unbleached
    or peroxide bleached when
    available)
Madura Tea
White vinegar (for cleaning)
Flyswat
Caring laundry powder and
    liquid, shampoos and
    deodorants, toilet soap

Chemist

Simple products

A to Z of Chemicals.
Available from Total Environment Centre, Argyle Street, Sydney. NSW

Atkinson, Russell Frank, *Your Health, Vitamins & Minerals* Doubleday, Australia 1982

Boericke, W., *Pocket Manual of Homoeopathic Materia Medica (complete manual of guiding symptoms of all remedies)* B. Jain Publishers PVT LTD. India 1984

Boyd, Hamish, *Introduction to Homoepathic Medicine* Keats Publishing Connecticut USA 1981

Buchman, Dian, *Feed Your Face*, Duckworth, London 1973

Buist, R., *Food Chemical Sensitivity* Harper & Row (Australasia) Pty Ltd. 1986

Carson, Rachel, *The Silent Spring* Houghton Mifflin, Boston 1962

Chancellor, Philip M., *Handbook of the Bach Flower Remedies* The C.W. Daniel Company Ltd, UK, 1971

Collison, David, *Why Do I Feel So Awful* Angus & Robertson Publishers, Sydney 1989

Gawler, Ian, *You Can Conquer Cancer* Hill of Content Publishing Company Pty Ltd, 1984

Gibson, D.M., *First Aid Homoeopathy in Accidents and Ailments*, India 1984

Grant, Doris & Joice, Jean, *Food Combining for Health* Thorsons, Wellingborough, UK 1984

Hanssen, Maurice *The New Additive Code Breaker* (Revised) Lothian Publishing Company Pty Ltd, Melbourne 1989

Hepper, Camilla, *Herbal Cosmetics* Thorsons, Wellingborough, UK 1987

* Mackarness, Richard, *Chemical Victims* Pan Books Ltd., London 1980

Madders, Jan, *Stress & Relaxation* Methuen, Australia 1983

Meares, Ainslie, *Relief Without Drugs* Fontana, Australia 1967

McMahon, Leonie, *Fatigue and how to beat it*, Macmillan, Australia, 1990.

Panos & Heimlich, *Homoeopathic Medicine at Home* Corgi, UK 1985

Sharma, *Homoeopathy & Natural Medicine* Thorsons, Wellingborough UK 1985

Shepherd, Dorothy, *Magic of the Minimum Dose* 1938 Health Science Press, Devon, UK 1938

Weeks, Nora, *The Medical Discoveries of Edward Bach, Physician* The C.W. Daniel Company Ltd, London 1940

Simply Living Vol 3 No. 9 'Water Filters' Page 82.

Choice May 1989 'Water Purifiers' Page 9.

Report to ME/CFS Society of NSW by Professor Denis Wakefield M.E. and YOU Newsletter January 1989.

'Pesticide Residues and the Stock Owner' (*Agfact* AO. 9.30, second edition, 1984) Authors: 1st Author Peter McGregor Regional Vet. Officer, Grafton, 2nd Author: Kerryn McDougall, Officer in Charge, Laboratory, Board of Tick Control, Lismore

'Chlorpyrifos in the Ambient Air of Houses Treated for Termites' C.G. Wright, R.B. Leidy, H.E. Dupree, Jr. *Bull. Environ. Contam. Toxicol,* (1988) Vol 40, Pages 561-568

NHRMC Report of the 1987 Market Basket Survey. Page 78.

IARC MONOGRAPHS Vol 40 Page 191.

* *Essential reading*

The information contained in this book I believe to be true and correct. I have always tried to obtain such information from the medical profession and technical personnel (with a knowledge of chemicals) employed by the various organisations, companies and firms; however, this has not always been possible. Therefore if there are any discrepancies please contact

Trixie Whitmore
PO Box 266
Pymble NSW 2073
or the publisher
Sally Milner Publishing Pty Ltd
17 Wharf Rd
Birchgrove 2041 Fax (02) 555 1463
so that the matter can be rectified in the next print run.